The Budget-Friendly
RENAL DIET COOKBOOK

Manage Chronic Kidney Disease and Avoid Dialysis with 100 Easy-to-Prepare, and Delicious Meals

ROWENA SAUNDERS, MS, RD, LDN

Dr. Lee Henton

Copyright © 2020 – Rowena Saunders

All rights reserved

No part of this publication may be reproduced, distributed, or transmitted in any form or by any means, including photocopying, recording, or other electronic or mechanical methods, without the prior written permission of the publisher, except in the case of brief quotations embodied in reviews and certain other non-commercial uses permitted by the United States copyright act of 1976.

Disclaimer

This publication is designed to provide reliable information on the subject matter only for educational purposes, and it is not intended to provide medical advice for any medical treatment. You should always consult your doctor or physician for guidance before you stop, start, or alter any nutrition prescriptions or attempt to implement the methods discussed. This book is published independently by the author and has no affiliation with any brands or products mentioned within it. The author hereby disclaims any responsibility or liability whatsoever that is incurred from the use or application of the contents of this

Contents

About The Author..10

Introduction..11

Chapter 1...15

Understanding Chronic Kidney Disease............................15

    How Kidneys Work in Our Body System.....................15

    Why Kidneys Are So Important......................................16

    What is Chronic Kidney Disease?....................................17

    Causes and Risk Factor of Chronic Kidney Disease......18

    Signs and Symptoms of Chronic Kidney Disease.........21

    Stages of Chronic Kidney Disease..................................23

Chapter 2...26

Diet and Kidney Disease Connection..................................26

    What is Renal Diet...26

    Foods to Eat and Limit or Avoid On a Renal Diet.........28

Chapter 3...44

Breakfast..44

publication by the purchaser or reader. The purchaser or reader is hereby liable for his or her own actions.

Zucchini Frittata..44

Egg Muffins...45

Strawberry Cottage Cheese Pancakes........................47

Mushroom and Red Pepper Omelet..........................49

Apple Fritter Rings..51

Gingerbread Muffins..52

French Toast and Cream Cheese with Applesauce.......54

Spaghetti-Basil Frittata...56

Berry Chia Pudding...57

Asparagus and Cheese Crepe Rolls..........................59

Breakfast Casserole...61

Grilled Corn and Cheesecakes (Arepas)....................62

German Pancakes..64

Homemade Turkey Sausage...................................65

Homemade Belgian Waffles...................................67

Chapter 4..70

Soups and Stew..70

Maryland Cream of Crab Soup...............................70

Rotisserie Chicken Noodle Soup.............................72

Irish Lamb Stew...74

Creamy Broccoli Soup..76

Southwestern Posole..78

Red Lentil Dahl...80

Shrimp and Crab Gumbo...82

Ground Beef Soup...84

Yucatan Chicken Lime Soup...86

Italian Wedding Soup..88

Beef and Barley Stew...91

Beef and Cabbage Borscht Soup...................................93

Seafood Corn Chowder Soup.......................................95

Spring Vegetable Soup...96

Chili Con Carne..98

Chapter 5...100

Snacks and Appetizers..100

Barbecue Meatballs..100

Hot Crab Dip..101

Lemonade Chicken Wings...103

Tortilla Rollups...104

Cinnamon Yogurt Fruit Dip.......................................106

Homemade Flour Tortilla Chips.................................108

Cucumber Cheese Sandwich Spread..........................109

Cold Veggie Pizza..110

Apple Filled Crepes...112

Apple Rice Salad...114

Fiesta Pinwheels...116

Brie with Cranberry Chutney...................................117

Lumpia Filipino Spring Rolls...................................119

Maple Trail Mix..122

Party Deviled Eggs..124

Chapter 6..126

Vegetables..126

Carrot Casserole...126

Zucchini French Fries...127

Marinated Fresh Vegetables....................................129

Ratatouille..131

Roasted Rosemary Cauliflower................................133

Seasoned Cabbage Steaks..134

Stuffed Zucchini Boats..135

Spanish Vegetable Paella...137

Yellow Hearty Squash Casserole..............................139

Bowtie Pasta with Veggie Crumbles and Kale..........141

Chapter 7..143

Seafood...143

Citrus Grilled Glazed Salmon...............................143

Maryland Crab Cakes...145

Tilapia Ceviche...147

Fish Tacos...148

Jambalaya...151

Asparagus Shrimp Linguini..................................152

Tuna Noodle Casserole...155

Oven-Fried Southern Style Catfish.......................156

Cilantro-Lime Cod..159

Shrimp Quesadilla..160

Chapter 8..163

Salad..163

Beet and Cucumber Salad.....................................163

Chicken Apple Crunch Salad................................164

Homestyle Macaroni Salad...................................166

Gelatin Salad with Cottage Cheese and Pineapple......167

Fruited Curry Chicken Salad................................168

Ambrosia Salad with Marshmallow.........................170

Rotini Pasta Salad...171

Spinach-Mandarin Salad..173

Turkey Waldorf Salad..174

Tabbouleh Salad..175

Chapter 9...178

Poultry and Meat Mains...178

Apple Spice Pork Chops..178

Beef Burritos...180

Herb-Roasted Pork Tenderloin................................181

Asian Orange Chicken...183

Garlic Chicken with Balsamic Vinegar.....................185

Turkey Breast with Cranberry Gravy.......................187

Grilled Pineapple Chicken.......................................189

Chicken Enchiladas...190

Roasted Leg of Lamb...192

Cranberry Pork Chops...194

Chapter 10...197

Dessert..197

Apple Pie Bars..197

Blueberry Peach Crisp……………………………………..199

Cherry Coffee Cake……………………………………….201

Fruity Peach Crisp Dump………………………………...202

Gingersnap Cookies………………………………………204

Lemon Icebox Pie…………………………………………205

Strawberry Pavlova……………………………………….207

Snickerdoodles……………………………………………209

Bread Pudding…………………………………………….210

Frozen Fruit Delight………………………………………212

Italian Tiramisu Cheesecake……………………………...214

Vanilla Lasagna…………………………………………...216

Lemon Yogurt Parfait…………………………………….217

Arroz Con Leche (Rice with Milk)………………………219

Bavarian Apple Torte…………………………………….220

Conclusion………………………………………………..223

About The Author

Rowena Saunders, MS, RD, LDN, is a registered and licensed dietitian and nutritionist with over 12 years of experience working as a food communications consultant in the health care and fitness/wellness industry in California, New York, Florida, and Texas. She completed and received her Bachelor's degree in Nutrition and Dietetics from Boston University, her master's degree in public health from the University of South Florida with a concentration in community and family health education, and completing her internship in Dietetic at the Oregon Health and Science University.

Rowena's areas of expertise are plant-based nutrition, natural organic eating, nutrition for wellness, disease prevention and management, disordered eating, sports and performance nutrition, and sustainable weight management.

Today, she focuses on providing food counseling to help her clients improve their food-body relationship in other to regain their health.

She enjoys cooking and having to spend time with family and friends.

Introduction

Being diagnosed with chronic kidney disease (CKD) is not the end of the world for you nor any affected member of your family, neither are you alone in this. Just so you know, about 37million adults in the US have been diagnosed with chronic kidney disease according to the Centers for Disease Control and Prevention (CDC), with about 1 in 10 people globally, and it is estimated that millions of people are at increased risk without even realizing it. Although CKD is not reversible, you can, however, prevent it from degenerating further. Studies show that only 1 out of 50 diagnosed with CKD end up undergoing dialysis treatment. In other words, early diagnosis and management can help stop the progression of the disease to kidney failure, thus prolonging your kidney function without the need for dialysis or kidney transplant. Managing CKD requires that you make certain necessary changes to your lifestyle habits, which, amongst others and undoubtedly one of the most critical changes, is your diet, which, according to the National Institute of Health (NIH), can slow the progression of CKD. One of the major concerns and fears most of my patients often express to me is having to give up their favorite foods for some tasteless diets in a bid to manage their CKD. But as an experienced and registered dietitian, I can assure you that would not be the case. You can eat foods that are not only delicious and nourishing, but that is also budget-friendly and healthy for your kidneys. Together, we can work not only to slow your CKD but ultimately prevent end-stage renal disease, dialysis, or kidney transplant through some modifications in your diet, which is aimed at controlling the amount of sodium, phosphorus, and potassium consumed.

In general, this book is designed to:

- Help you manage your CKD non-dialysis with handpicked renal diet meals that are not only low in sodium, potassium, and phosphorus but also delicious with easy-to-follow recipes and graphical images to complement each meal
- Provide dietary choices and recommendations that accommodate people with end-stage renal disease or people on dialysis treatment as well as those with diabetes
- Provide you with quick tips you can adapt to modify certain recipe to suit your specific dietary needs

- Provide you with the nutritional information of each meal servings, as well as the recommended serving size to help you measure the quantity to be served in other to stay within the prescribed nutrient limit
- Educate you on certain dietary information needed to make the best meal preparation decisions such as foods low and high in sodium, potassium, and phosphorus
- Provide you with the number of ingredients necessary to make calculated decisions when mapping out your daily meal plans.

…And much more

At first, adopting a kidney-friendly diet can be quite challenging due to your unpreparedness in dietary changes from what you are used to, and to top it off, you may be dealing with diabetes alongside CKD, calling for even stricter food restrictions. However, carefully following the recipes with the additional tips outlined in this book will help reduce the anxiety you may feel when faced with selecting the right food options for your everyday life. I have seen many of my patients overcome the fears that came after being diagnosed with CKD while going on to live a happy and healthy life with functional kidneys all from the knowledge shared in this book. This, too, can be you, and I hope and believe that the pages of this book would inspire and educate you enough to alter the trajectory of your health for the better.

So, without further ado, let's begin proper.

Chapter 1

Understanding Chronic Kidney Disease

Chronic Kidney disease, also called renal disease, is the general term that describes the reduction of kidney function, which is estimated to have affected about 10 percent of the world's population. Being diagnosed with CKD does not imply a kidney failure or the need for a kidney transplant. For what its worth, CKD is a manageable disease which, when detected early, can be prevented from further degeneration through certain changes in your lifestyle, most importantly, your diet, which is the core focus of this book. But before we get to your dietary changes, I would briefly shed some light on how the kidney works, and what you need to know about chronic kidney disease.

So, let's get started.

How Kidneys Work in Our Body System

The kidneys are a two bean-shaped organ located just below your rib cage with each kidney positioned on the sides of your spine. At about a million functioning units called nephrons are contained in each kidney. A nephron, on the other hand, is made up of a filtering unit called glomerulus (small blood vessels attached to a tubule). When blood enters the glomerulus, it gets filtered, with the remainder of the fluid passing along the tubule. In the tubule, chemicals and water are either added or removed from the filtered fluid (based on the needs of the body) to make urine. This urine then flows to the bladder via the ureters (two thin tubes of muscle), with each positioned on the sides of your bladder. The urine is stored in the bladder between 1—8hours before it is excreted. Your kidneys, ureters, and bladder form the major part of your urinary tract.

Why Kidneys Are So Important

Most of us know that one significant role of the kidneys in our body is the removal of waste products and excess fluid through urine, which is essential in maintaining a balance of body chemicals. However, the importance of the kidneys goes beyond the removal of wastes and excess fluid; the kidneys also ensures the critical regulation of our body from potassium, body's salt, and acid content. The kidneys are also responsible for producing hormones that impact the function of other organs. For example, the erythropoietin (EPO) hormone, which is produced by the kidney, stimulates the production of red blood cells by the bone marrow. It is also responsible for stimulating the production of the renin hormone, which helps in blood pressure regulation.

Other functions performed by the kidneys are:

- Balancing and maintaining the overall fluids in the body
- Filtering wastes from food, toxic substances, and drugs
- Production of vitamin D for strong, healthy bones
- Regulating the levels of pH, potassium, and salt in the body.

As you have seen, the role of the kidneys is essential to the functioning of important processes that our body undergoes. In the following sections, I would through more light on what could go wrong with the kidney, the implications of a malfunctioning kidney, and how it can be managed and prevented from resulting in treatment by dialysis or kidney transplant.

What is Chronic Kidney Disease?

Chronic kidney disease (CKD) occurs when your kidneys become damaged and unable to perform its functions to full capacity for more than three months. In its early stage (stage 1-3), you may notice little to no symptoms, which is easier to treat if it is detected on time. However, when it gets to an advanced stage (stage 4-5), it can lead to the build-up of dangerous levels of fluid and wastes in your body, resulting to swelling in the arms and legs, high blood pressure, weak bones, decreased immune response, inability to concentrate, erectile dysfunction and cardiovascular disease among many others. CKD is in stages, and the stage of kidney disease is determined by the glomerular filtration rate (GFR) – a test that measures the level of a kidney function and the stage of CKD.

CKD not properly managed would get worse over time and would ultimately result in kidney failure. When this happens, treatment options must be sought after to survive, such as dialysis or a kidney transplant, else death becomes inevitable. With that being said, the goal is not to allow the disease to degenerate into a kidney failure but to help you best manage the condition by slowing its progression and keeping your kidneys up and running for as long as possible. Your choice of diet most especially can accelerate the progression of CKD, resulting in kidney failure. The diet section of this book is aimed at helping you manage your CKD without having to put your kidneys at risk of failure.

Causes and Risk Factor of Chronic Kidney Disease

The conditions or diseases that primarily causes CKD include:

Diabetes (Type 1 and 2)

Diabetes occurs when the body is unable to produce enough insulin to control blood sugar (Type 1) or cannot properly use insulin to control blood sugar (Type 2), either of which results in a high blood sugar level. Over time, the increased sugar level in the blood would damage the kidney's tiny filtering units of small blood vessels (glomeruli). This damage then disrupts the filtering of wastes from the blood, thereby resulting in kidney disease and, eventually, kidney failure if uncontrolled. In the US, diabetes is responsible for about 44% of kidney disease and is the number one cause of kidney failure.

High blood pressure

High blood pressure (hypertension) is another major cause of kidney disease and other health complications, e.g., heart attacks and strokes. High blood pressure is when the force of blood against the walls of your artery (helps convey blood from the heart to all parts of the body) increases. When it does, it also increases the pressure in the glomeruli, thereby making the kidney to lose its ability to function. In the US, high blood pressure accounts for about 29% cause of kidney failure and is the second leading cause of kidney failure in the US after diabetes.

Glomerular disease

When the glomeruli are unable to play its role in the kidney, it is called a glomeruli disease. This disease is specifically called glomerulonephritis and is responsible for the inflammation of the glomeruli – which it does by damaging the kidney's filter system so that the kidneys are not able to filter waste and fluid properly.

Polycystic kidney disease

Polycystic kidney disease is, by far, the most common inherited kidney disease that is passed down through families. The characterization of this disease is such that when kidney cysts are formed and enlarges over a period of time, it causes the expansion of the kidney and its inability to function, resulting in kidney damage. Other diseases passed down through families that can affect the kidneys are Alport's syndrome, primary hyperoxaluria, and cystinuria.

Other conditions that can cause kidney disease are:

- Urinary tract infections
- Kidney stones
- Interstitial nephritis, i.e., an inflammation of the kidney's tubules

- Vesicoureteral reflux, i.e., a condition that causes urine to go back up into your kidneys

In addition to the common causes of CKD identified above, you are still at risk of the disease if you fall under any one of the following risk factors:

- A history of kidney disease in your family
- Old age especially from age 50
- Heart and blood vessel (cardiovascular) disease
- Smoking
- Obesity
- Overuse of painkiller medications that contain naproxen, ibuprofen, or acetaminophen
- Chronic use of street drugs, i.e., heroin and crack
- Certain ethnicities, i.e., African-American, Native American, or Hispanic, are more prone to high blood pressure and diabetes, which can cause kidney disease.

Signs and Symptoms of Chronic Kidney Disease

The signs and symptoms of CKD often occur late, much after the condition has progressed. CKD is sometimes called a "silent" condition; this is because it is difficult to detect, especially most people with early-stage CKD. While being on the lookout for late-stage symptoms would not help with early detection, it is still important that you're aware of the signs. Nonetheless, for early detection of CKD, you mustn't wait for the symptoms to manifest before taking necessary actions. If you are at risk of CKD, immediately get yourself tested, and it should be done at least once a year or per the instructions of your doctor. The earlier the detection of CKD, the greater the benefit that comes from early treatment.

It is essential to see a doctor and get tested should you observe any of the signs and symptoms of CKD below:

- Changes in urination such as more or less urine than usual, bloody or foamy urine, or waking up more often at night to urinate
- Fatigue and weakness
- Continuous itching
- Swelling in hands or feet
- Shortness of breath
- Chest pain
- Poor appetite
- Nausea
- Vomiting
- Puffiness around the eyes, especially in the morning
- Sleep problems

- Reduced mental sharpness
- Muscle cramps

Bear in mind that these signs and symptoms are often nonspecific, implying that other illnesses can cause them. However, its better safe than sorry by being proactive and getting tested if you notice any of the above signs and symptoms.

Stages of Chronic Kidney Disease

In February 2002, the National Kidney Foundation (NKF) released a guideline to assist medical practitioners in classifying the stage of CKD. The stages of CKD were classified into five. Being able to identify the stage of kidney disease helps medical practitioners to be able to proffer the best medical treatment, given that each stage requires a different treatment option.

For each stage of kidney disease to be understood, we must first understand how to measure the level of kidney function. The universally accepted standard of measurement of a kidney function is the Glomerular Filtration Rate (GFR), which measures the effectiveness of your kidneys and how well it filters wastes and fluids from your blood. Each stage of kidney disease corresponds to a GFR range, which is determined upon conducting a test. One such common test is the serum creatinine test, which determines the level of creatinine in the blood. GFR is then calculated using a pre-defined medical equation, which would require the result from the serum creatinine test, including other parameters such as age, race, weight, body size, and gender. Other tests that can be performed to determine the level of your kidney function include kidney biopsy, CT scan, and urine test.

Stages	GFR (mL/min)	Description	Likely Signs and Symptoms
Stage 1	90 or higher	Kidney damage but with a normal kidney function	High blood pressure, swelling in legs, urinary tract infections or abnormal urine test
Stage 2	60-89	Mild loss of kidney function	
Stage 3	3a: 45-59 3b: 30-44	3a: Mild to moderate loss of kidney function 3b: Moderate to a severe loss of kidney	Low blood count, malnutrition, bone pain, unusual pain, numbness or tingling, decreased mental sharpness or feeling unwell

		function	
Stage 4	15-29	Severe loss of kidney function	Anemia, decreased appetite, bone disease or abnormal blood levels of phosphorus, calcium or vitamin D
Stage 5 or end-stage renal disease	Less than 15	Kidney failure with a need for transplant or dialysis	Uremia, fatigue, shortness of breath, nausea, vomiting, abnormal thyroid levels, swelling in hands/legs/eyes/lower back or lower back pain

While it is essential to see a doctor and get tested if you observe any of the signs and symptoms of CKD already discussed, you should do the same if you fall under any of the causes and risk factors associated with CKD. This would help you know your GFR and at what stage of kidney disease you belong to – ultimately enabling you to make informed decisions regarding the health of your kidney as well as keeping your kidneys up and running for long, without degenerating to end-stage renal disease.

Chapter 2

Diet and Kidney Disease Connection

To effectively manage CKD, lifestyle changes (regular exercise, weight management, avoiding smoking cigarettes, non-use of alcohol, etc.), working with health care providers, and changes in your diet are of paramount importance. That being said, adopting a kidney-friendly diet is one of the most important ways to manage CKD. When you are in the early stage of CKD (stage 1-3), some changes would need to be made to your diet to prevent the disease from degenerating further. This would require you to limit your intake of potassium, phosphorous, sodium, and protein. However, if the disease becomes advanced (stage 4-5), you would have to follow through with stricter alterations to your diet. Not adhering to the right amount of nutrients and minerals in your diet may result in the build-up of wastes and the inability of your kidneys to remove such from your blood effectively, thereby exacerbating the kidney disease, which can lead to kidney failure if left uncontrolled.

What is Renal Diet

A renal diet is prescribed for someone with kidney disease, and this prescription is based on the stage of kidney disease, blood work results, and if there is a presence of diabetes or high blood pressure. There is no standard renal diet prescription, given that diet prescription varies between persons. However, the goal of a renal diet is:

- To prevent the build-up of wastes in the blood as well as the complications that can arise from waste build-up, e.g., risk of cardiovascular disease
- To slow the progression of chronic kidney disease and reduce the kidneys workload (before dialysis occurs)
- To maintain maximum nutritional needs and prevent the loss of lean body mass.

While renal diet may vary from person to person, the common themes of nutrients and minerals to be mindful of are sodium, potassium, phosphorus, protein, and fluids. Everyone is different; therefore, each person would need to be guided by a dietitian to come up with a renal diet tailored to the individual's needs. In subsequent sections, I would be revealing some recommended, handpicked diets that meet the criteria of the right amount of renal diet nutrients and minerals that you can start off with right away.

Foods to Eat and Limit or Avoid On a Renal Diet

Eating the right food is all about keeping your kidney disease under control. While it is important to generally maintain a healthy food diet such as watching your intake of calories, fats, and carbohydrates, it is more important especially if you have chronic kidney disease to be mindful of certain foods that have a high amount of the common themes of nutrients and minerals (as earlier mentioned). Below, I discuss briefly on these nutrients and minerals, as well as some foods that should be limited (if the intake of nutrient and mineral content are well-controlled) or avoided and foods that should be included in your diet.

Sodium

Sodium is a mineral mostly contained in most foods and helps balance the amount of fluid in the body. Most people commonly interchange salt with sodium and vice versa. The common salt (table salt) is made up of sodium and chloride, and it is the sodium in the salt (about 40%) that is bad for your health. Although salt is the major source of sodium in our diet, it is not the only source. Other sources of sodium in our foods are

- Sodium sulfite: Used for preventing discoloration of dried fruits
- Sodium alginate: Used in chocolate milk and ice-cream

- Sodium benzoate: Used as a preservative in sauce
- Sodium citrate: Used for flavor enhancement in gelatin, desserts and beverages
- Sodium bicarbonate: Used as soda and baking powder
- Sodium nitrate: Used for the preservation and coloration of processed meat
- Sodium saccharide: Used as an artificial sweetener

Healthy kidneys are well able to regulate the excess sodium present in the body. However, having excess sodium in the body is harmful to people with kidney disease. Because sodium attracts water, excess intake of sodium would result in retention of fluid in the body, and when this occurs, the kidneys become unable to discharge the excess sodium and fluid effectively. As sodium and fluid build-ups in the body of people with CKD, it may lead to:

- Increased thirst
- Swellings in the leg, hand, and face
- High blood pressure
- Heart failure and,
- Shortness of breath

It is recommended that CKD patients should consume less than 2000mg of sodium per day (preferably about 1500mg). Therefore, it is increasingly important that you monitor your sodium intake. You should, for instance:

- Limit or avoid foods with high sodium, and if you must have vegetable foods that are high in sodium, then you must reduce the amount of sodium by boiling, and throwing away its water.
- Restrict salt intake and cook food without salt. If salt reduces the flavor in your food, use spices and condiments that do not list salt in its title for that extra flavor, e.g., choose garlic powder or onion powder rather than garlic salt or onion salt.
- Always read food labels and look out not only for salt but also for other compounds that contain sodium. Check the labels and choose "sodium-free" or "low-sodium" products. However, ensure potassium isn't used as a substitute for sodium in these foods.
- Pay attention to the serving size.
- Compare labels of similar products with the same servings and choose that with the lowest in sodium.
- Eat more home-made food as they tend to have lesser sodium when cooked from scratch than most instant and boxed mixes.

Below are some high sodium foods to limit or avoid and low sodium foods you should incorporate in your diet.

Meats, Poultry, Fish, Legumes, Eggs, and Nuts	
High Sodium Foods	Low Sodium Foods
Smoked, salted, canned or processed meat, fish or poultry which includes bacon, frankfurters, sausage, ham, sardines, and caviar	Eggs and its substitutes
Frozen breaded meats, e.g., burritos	Peanut butter with low sodium
Canned entrees, e.g., spam, chili, and ravioli	Beans and dry peas (not canned)
Salted nuts	Canned fish or poultry with its water or oil drained
Canned beans with salt added	

Dairy Products	
High Sodium Foods	Low Sodium Foods
Buttermilk	Milk, ice cream, yogurt, and ice milk
Processed cheese, sauces and cheese spreads	Cheeses, ricotta cheese and mozzarella with low sodium

Bread, Grains, and Cereals	
High Sodium Foods	Low Sodium Foods
Bread and rolls with salt added to its tops	Bread, rolls, and bagels with no salt added to its tops
Quick bread, and biscuit	Muffins
Pizza, salted crackers, croutons	Rice and pasta with no salt added when cooking

Processed mixes for potatoes, pasta, and rice	Corn, noodles, and flour tortillas with low sodium
	Popcorn, pretzels, and chips without salt

Vegetables and Fruits

High Sodium Foods	Low Sodium Foods
Regular vegetable juices and canned vegetables	Frozen and fresh vegetables with no sauce
Olives, sauerkraut, and pickles	Tomato or V-8 juice with low salt
Vegetables prepared with bacon, ham, or salted pork	Fresh fruit
Packaged mixes, e.g., tater tots and frozen hash browns.	Dried fruits
Pasta, salsa, and tomato sauces prepared commercially	Frozen vegetables

Soups

High Sodium Foods	Low Sodium Foods
Regular canned and dehydrated soup, bouillon, and broth	Canned and dehydrated soups, bouillon, and broth with low sodium
Seasoned ramen mixes	Unsalted home-made soups

Fats, Desserts, and Sweets

High Sodium Foods	Low Sodium Foods

Soy sauce, ketchup, BBQ sauce, and marinara sauce	Vinegar, butter or margarine with no salt
Regular salad dressing with bacon bits and bottled salad dressings	Vegetable oils, and salad dressings and sauces with low sodium
Margarine or salted butter	Mayonnaise
Cake and instant pudding	All unsalted desserts

Potassium

Potassium, just like sodium, is contained in most foods we eat, and it is also found naturally in the body. Potassium helps to keep a regular heartbeat and ensures the muscles are working as it should. It is also necessary for maintaining the balance of fluid and electrolyte in the bloodstream. Healthy kidneys keep the right amount of potassium in the body while it discharges excess amounts of it into the urine.

Having excess potassium in the body is unhealthy for people with CKD. This is because their kidneys are unable to expel the excess potassium, causing a build-up of potassium levels in the body. High levels of potassium in the blood are called hyperkalemia, and this can cause:

- Weakness in muscles
- Irregular heartbeat
- Slow pulse
- Heart attacks and;
- Death

People with CKD are to limit their total potassium intake to between 1500mg and 2000mg per day. Nonetheless, your dietitian or physician will be in the best position to advise you on the precise restriction level based on the state of health of your kidneys. Personal measures should also be taken to monitor your potassium intake. You should take note of the following:

- Limit or avoid foods high in potassium, and if you must have vegetable foods that are high in potassium, then you must reduce the amount of potassium. To do this, peel and cut the vegetables into smaller pieces, soak for at least 5 hours or more, rinse with warm water, then boil and discard the water
- Don't use or drink canned fruits and vegetable liquids or the juices from cooked meat.
- All foods contain some amount of potassium. Hence, choose foods with low potassium when possible and be mindful of the serving size. Remember this; eating a large amount of low

potassium food is the same as eating a high potassium food.
- Your physician or doctor should conduct a periodic test (once a month) on your blood potassium levels.

Below are some high potassium foods to limit or avoid and low potassium foods you should incorporate in your diet.

Fruits	
High Potassium Foods	**Low Potassium Foods**
Avocado	Apple Juice
Apricot	Apple
Banana	Apple sauce
Cantaloupe	Blackberries
Dates	Blueberries
Dried figs	Cherries
Grapefruit Juice	Cranberries
Honeydew	Fruit Cocktail
Kiwi	Grapes
Mango	Grape Juice
Nectarine	Grapefruit
Orange	Mandarin Oranges
Orange Juice	Pineapple
Papaya	Pineapple Juice
Pomegranate	Plums
Pomegranate Juice	Raspberries
Prunes	Strawberries
Prune Juice	Tangerine
Guava	Watermelon
Vegetables	

High Potassium Foods	Low Potassium Foods
Acorn Squash	Alfalfa sprouts
Artichoke	Asparagus
Bamboo Shoots	Green or wax bean Raw or cooked broccoli from frozen
Baked Beans	Cabbage Red and green carrots
Butternut Squash	Cauliflower
Refried beans	Celery
Fresh then boiled beets	Fresh corn
Red and black beans	Cucumber
Potato	Eggplant
Brussels sprouts	Kale
Chinese cabbage	Lettuce
Raw carrots	Mixed vegetables
Dried beans and peas	Raw white mushrooms
Greens excluding kale	Onions
Hubbard Squash	Parsley
Kohlrabi	Green peas
Sweet potato	Peppers
Legumes	Radish
Cooked white mushrooms	Rhubarb
Okra	Canned water chestnut
Parsnips	Watercress
White and sweet potatoes	Yellow squash
Pumpkin	Zucchini squash
Other Foods	
High Potassium Foods	Low Potassium Foods
Chocolate	Rice
Granola	Noodles
Nuts and seeds	Pasta
Peanut butter	Bread (not whole grain)
Lona salt (salt substitute)	Angel and yellow cake

Potato chips	Canned tuna
Chocolate cakes	Pies with no chocolate
Snuff or chewing tobacco	Cookies with no chocolate or nuts
Chocolate ice cream	Turkey (white meat)

Phosphorus

Phosphorus, which is found in most foods, is a mineral that works with calcium for bone development and maintenance. Phosphorus also helps in developing organs and connective tissues as well as aiding muscle movement. Healthy kidneys can maintain the right amount of phosphorous in your blood and expel excess phosphorus. When kidney function is impaired or if you have CKD (especially at stage 4-5), your kidneys become unable to remove excess phosphorus. A high amount of phosphorus in your blood can cause the calcium in your bones to be removed, thus resulting in weak bones. This can also lead to the harmful deposit of calcium in your blood vessels, heart, lungs, and eyes with an increased risk of heart attack, stroke, or death. For people with CKD, your total phosphorus intake should be restricted to about 800 and 1000 mg per day.

Below are general measures to take in other to control your phosphorus intake

- Phosphorous is found in foods that are rich in protein; thus, eat proteinaceous foods that are low in phosphorous.
- Discuss with your physician or doctor about using phosphate binders during mealtime. Phosphate binders are medications that help reduce the absorption of phosphate in foods, and often taken by people with CKD who are unable to discharge excess phosphate from their body
- Avoid processed foods that have additives or preservatives (inorganic phosphorus). Look for phosphorus or "PHOS" on the label of ingredients

Below is a list of foods that has high phosphorous content as well as foods with low phosphorus alternatives:

High Phosphorus Foods	Low Phosphorus Foods
Fast foods, convenience foods, and gas station foods	Home-cooked meals or snacks prepared using fresh ingredients
Soy milk, and enriched milk	Unenriched almond or rice milk
Cheese spreads and processed cheeses	A small portion of brie or swiss cheese
Fat-free sour cream or fat-free cream cheese	Low or regular sour cream or fat cream cheese
Frozen yogurt or ice cream or	Sherbet, frozen fruit pops or sorbet
Quick bread, biscuits,	Fresh dinner rolls, bagels,

cornbread	bread or English muffins
Processed meats, e.g., bacon, chicken nuggets, bologna, ham and hot dogs, including meat, poultry or seafood that has "phos" in its label of ingredients	Lean beef, lamb, eggs or natural seafood, poultry or any other fish with no "phos" in its label of ingredients
Chocolate or caramel which included candy bars and chocolate drinks	Jelly beans, fruit snacks, hard candy or gumdrops
Pepper-type sodas, colas, and some flavored waters, energy or sports drinks, bottled teas, beer, wine, and some drink mixes that has "phos" in its label of ingredients	Lemon-lime soda, root beer, plain water, ginger ale and some drink mixes (without "phos" in its label), brewed coffee (fresh and made from beans) or brewed tea (from tea bags)

The image below is a sample food label with quick guides to the left on how to interprete food labels.

Serving Size –
Always look here first.
Sodium Goal:
2000 mg a day
600 mg a meal
100 - 200 mg a snack

Sodium –
Always look at the "**mg**" and **NOT** the "**%**"!

Ingredient List –
Look for *phosphorus* or words with "**phos**" in them.

Phosphoric Acid
Hexametaphosphate
Dicalcium Phosphate
Monocalcium Phosphate
Tricalcium Phosphate
Sodium Phosphate

Stay away from added phosphorus! It adds up to 1000mg phosphorus per day.

Ingredients: Ground Corn Treated with Lime, Water, Cellulose Gum, Propionic Acid (to preserve freshness), Benzoic Acid (to preserve freshness), Phosphoric Acid (preservative), Dextrose, Guar Gum, Amylase.

Potassium – listing is not required.
No listing does **NOT** mean no potassium.

Nutrition Facts

Serving Size 2 tortillas (51g)
Serving Per Container 6

Amount Per Serving
Calories 110   Calories from Fat 10

	% Daily Value*
Total Fat 1g	2%
Saturated Fat 0g	0%
Trans Fat 0g	
Cholesterol 0mg	0%
Sodium 30mg	1%
Total Carbohydrate 22g	7%
Dietary Fiber 2g	9%
Sugar 0g	
Protein 2g	

Vitamin A 0%	*	Vitamin C 0%
Calcium 2%	*	Iron 4%

*Percent Daily Values are based on a 2,000 calorie diet. Your daily values may be higher or lower depending on your calorie needs:

	Calories	2,000	2,500
Total Fat	Less than	65g	80g
Saturated Fat	Less than	20g	25g
Cholesterol	Less than	300mg	300mg
Sodium	Less than	2,400mg	2,400mg
Total Carbohydrate		300g	375g
Dietary Fiber		25g	30g

Calories per gram:
Fat 9 * Carbohydrate 4 * Protein 4

If your food has the Daily Value listed for phosphorus, use this guide:

0% - 5% Daily Value – Low phosphorus (0-50 mg)

5% - 15% Daily Value – Medium phosphorus (51-150 mg)

Over 15% Daily Value – High phosphorus (150 mg or higher)

Protein

Protein is an essential nutrient that helps in repairing tissues, building muscles, and fighting infections, among other bodily functions. Having protein in the bloodstream is not a problem for healthy kidneys because when it is ingested, waste products are formed, which is then filtered and turned into urine. In contrast, impaired kidneys are unable to expel protein waste, which then accumulates in the blood. The more protein waste is accumulated, and that needs to be removed, the more difficult it is for the kidneys to get rid of it. This can stress out your kidneys, causing them to degenerate even faster. The right amount of protein consumption is thus very essential but also tricky for CKD patients; this is because the amount differs depending on the stage of the disease, and the body size of the patient and too little protein can result in malnutrition. Hence, you must consume the recommended amount for the exact stage of the disease based on the advice of your dietitian. For people with CKD who are not on dialysis, a diet that is low in protein is recommended. It is suggested by many studies that if you want to limit the amount of protein intake, including plant-based foods in your diet is a great way to go about it. This is because plant-based foods naturally contain less protein than animal-based foods and can help slow the progression of damage in kidney function.

It is recommended that people with stage 1-2 CKD non-dialysis should eat 0.8 grams of protein daily per kilogram of ideal body weight and 0.55-0.6 grams of protein for stage 3-4 CKD non-dialysis. On the other hand, if you are on dialysis, the amount of protein intake needs to be increased because when waste is filtered from your blood, it also expels protein, and when there is not enough protein in your blood, your body will use the proteins in your muscles for what it needs. This can subject you to infections, cause you to lose weight, and make you feel tired. People on dialysis treatment (stage 5 CKD) are recommended to eat about 1-1.2 grams of protein per kilogram of ideal body weight each day.

Fluids

We all need water to survive; however, when a person has CKD, the amount consumed needs to be controlled. This is because impaired kidneys are unable to discharge excess fluid from the body. Excess fluid in the body of CKD patients is dangerous and can result in high blood pressure and heart failure. Excess fluid can likewise build-up in the lungs, making it difficult to breathe, especially with people on dialysis treatment. Depending on the stage of your CKD and treatment, your physician or doctor may advise you to cut back on your fluid intake. The amount of fluid intake is individualized, depending on urine output and other factors. You must adhere to your doctor's fluid intake guidelines. Also, you may need to cut down foods with high water content, limit sodium intake to avoid being thirsty, and be mindful of the amount of water used in cooking.

Having had a good understanding of the renal diet guidelines per our earlier discussions on the common themes of nutrients, I now suppose you have a fair idea of what type of foods to include in your diet and foods to avoid or restrict. In subsequent sections, I have carefully handpicked certain low budget and kidney-friendly meals that you can easily prepare and include as part of your renal diet irrespective of your CKD stage, whether you are on dialysis or whether you have diabetes.

Chapter 3

Breakfast

Zucchini Frittata

Suitable For: CKD non-dialysis, dialysis, and diabetes

Preparation Time: 10 minutes; **Cooking Time**: 35 minutes; **Servings**: 9; **Serving Size**: 3⅔ x 2⅓-inch piece

Ingredients:

- ¼ cup of chopped parsley
- 3 cups of grated zucchini
- 1 medium-sized chopped onion
- 1 clove of minced garlic
- ½ cup of canola oil
- ½ cup of grated parmesan cheese
- ½ teaspoon of dried marjoram
- 4 large eggs, slightly beaten
- 1 cup of Bisquick baking mix
- Pepper to taste

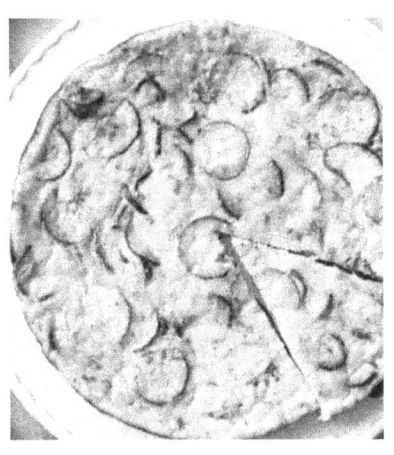

Directions:

1. Preheat the oven to 350° F

2. Combine and mix all ingredients in a large bowl
3. Pour mixed ingredients into a greased pan of 11 x 7-inch, then bake for about 35 minutes until it becomes light brown
4. Cut in 9 pieces and serve

Nutrients Per Serving: Calories 230, Protein 6g, Carbohydrates 11g, Fat 18g, Cholesterol 98mg, Sodium 260mg, Potassium 198mg, Phosphorus 107mg, Fiber 1.1g

Tips:

1. Leftovers still taste lovely. Simply refrigerate and reheat in the oven when next you want to have your Zucchini

Egg Muffins

Suitable For: CKD non-dialysis, dialysis, and diabetes

Preparation Time: 15 minutes; **Cooking Time:** 22 minutes; **Servings:** 8; **Serving Size:** 1 muffin

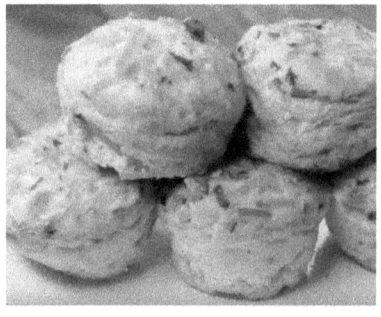

Ingredients:

- 1 cup of bell peppers (yellow, red, and orange)
- 1 cup of onion

- ½ pound of ground pork
- ¼ teaspoon of poultry seasoning
- ¼ teaspoon of garlic powder
- ¼ teaspoon of onion powder
- ½ teaspoon of Mrs. Dash herb seasoning
- 8 large eggs
- 2 tablespoons of milk or its substitute

Directions:

1. Preheat the oven to 350° F and spray a muffin tin of regular size with cooking spray.
2. Dice the bell peppers and onion.
3. Combine pork, garlic powder, poultry seasoning, onion powder, and Mrs. Dash seasoning in a bowl to make sausage.
4. Cook the sausage crumbles in a non-stick skillet until it is ready, then drain.
5. Use the milk or its substitute to beat eggs.
6. Add and mix the sausage crumbles and vegetables.
7. Pour the mixed egg into the prepared muffin tins, then allow the muffins to rise. Bake for 22 minutes.

Nutrients Per Serving: Calories 154, Protein 12g, Carbohydrates 3g, Fat 10g, Cholesterol 230mg, Sodium 155mg, Potassium 200mg, Phosphorus 154mg, Fiber 0.5g

Tips:

- For a quick breakfast entrée, refrigerate leftover muffins and reheat for 30-40 seconds in the oven
- The size of a regular muffin tin cup holds 3½ ounces. If you desire, use a smaller muffin tin; however, the cooking time should be reduced

Strawberry Cottage Cheese Pancakes

Suitable For: CKD non-dialysis, dialysis, and diabetes

Preparation Time: 5 minutes; **Cooking Time:** 10 minutes; **Servings:** 6; **Serving Size:** Two 4-inch pancakes

Ingredients:

- 1 cup of cottage cheese
- 4 eggs, slightly beaten
- ½ cup of all-purpose white flour
- 6 tablespoons of melted unsalted butter
- Non-stick cooking spray
- 3 cups of fresh strawberries, sliced

Directions:

1. Combine the cottage cheese, eggs, flour and butter

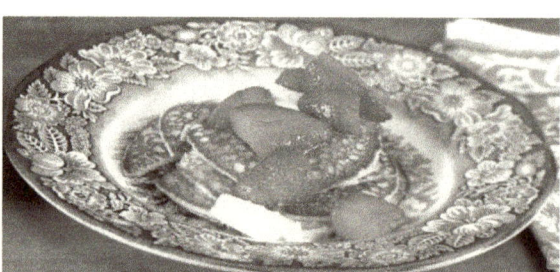

in a medium-sized bowl
2. Spray griddle or frying pan using a non-stick cooking spray
3. Heat the griddle or frying pan over medium-high heat, and pour about ¼ cup of the mixed cottage cheese onto the griddle or frying pan to form pancakes
4. Allow pancakes to cook for about 2-3 minutes until it becomes lightly browned on the undersides. Turn to the other side and have it lightly browned
5. Remove the pancakes and place in a heated platter
6. Use the remaining mixed cottage cheese to make additional pancakes
7. Serve each pancake and top with ½ cup of sliced strawberries

Nutrients Per Serving: Calories 253, Protein 11g, Carbohydrates 21g, Fat 17g, Cholesterol 182mg, Sodium 172mg, Potassium 217mg, Phosphorus 159mg, Fiber 2.0g

Tips:

- Raspberries, blackberries, blueberries, or peaches (canned) can be used as a substitute for strawberries

- Pancakes can likewise be topped with a regular or sugar-free jam or pancake syrup

Mushroom and Red Pepper Omelet

Suitable For: CKD non-dialysis, dialysis, and diabetes

Preparation Time: 5 minutes; **Cooking Time:** 10 minutes; **Servings:** 2; **Serving Size:** ½ omelet

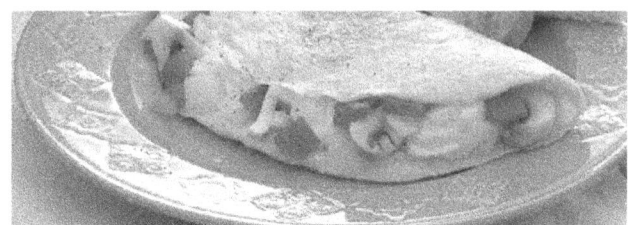

Ingredients:

- ½ cup of raw mushroom pieces
- 2 tablespoons of onion
- ¼ cup of canned sweet red peppers
- 2 teaspoons of unsalted butter
- 3 large eggs
- 1 teaspoon of Worcestershire sauce
- 2 tablespoons of whipped cream cheese
- ¼ teaspoon of black pepper

Directions:

1. Dice the mushrooms, red peppers, and onion

2. Use a skillset and melt one teaspoon of the butter over medium heat, then add the mushrooms and onion. Sauté for about 5 minutes until the onion becomes tender. Add the diced pepper and stir. Remove the vegetables from the skillet and put aside
3. In the skillet, melt the leftover teaspoon of butter. Using the Worcestershire sauce, beat the eggs and cook over medium heat.
4. When the eggs have been partially cooked, add the vegetable mixture, and place the whipped cream cheese over the vegetables. Evenly cook the undersides of the omelet until the eggs are set
5. Remove skillet from heat, fold omelet into half, then use the black pepper to sprinkle the omelet.

Nutrients Per Serving: Calories 199, Protein 11g, Carbohydrates 4g, Fat 15g, Cholesterol 341mg, Sodium 276mg, Potassium 228mg, Phosphorus 167mg, Fiber 0.6g

Tips:

- The Sautéed onion will not be brown when cooked but will appear transparent
- Use non-stick skillet or cooking spray to reduce the amount of fat, use trans-fat free margarine (if you desire) in place of unsalted butter, and use low cholesterol egg as substitute rather than whole eggs

Apple Fritter Rings

Suitable For: CKD non-dialysis, dialysis, and diabetes

Preparation Time: 10 minutes; **Cooking Time:** 25 minutes; **Servings:** 20; **Serving Size:** 1 fritter

Ingredients:

- 4 large tart cooking apples
- 1 cup of all-purpose white flour
- 6 tablespoons of sugar (divided use)
- 1 teaspoon of baking powder
- 1 large beaten egg
- ⅓ cup of low-fat milk
- ⅓ cup of almond milk
- 1 teaspoon of canola oil
- ¾ cup of oil for deep-fat frying
- ½ teaspoon of cinnamon

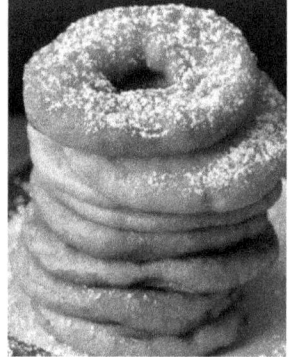

Directions:

1. Peel and core the apples, cutting each into five rings, approximately ½-inch thick
2. Altogether, sift the flour, two tablespoons of sugar and baking powder in a mixing bowl
3. Combine and mix the egg, milk, almond milk and one teaspoon of oil in a separate bowl

4. Add the egg mixture to the dry ingredients from step 1 and stir until it blends
5. Using a skillet of about 2-inch deep, heat 1-inch cooking oil to 375º F
6. Dip the slices of apple into the batter one at a time, and fry in the hot oil for about 1½ minutes or until it is golden brown. Drain on paper towels
7. Combine the remaining ¼ cup of /sugar with the cinnamon, sprinkling over the fritters. Serve hot

Nutrients Per Serving: Calories 145, Protein 1g, Carbohydrates 15g, Fibre 1.3g, Fat 9g, Sodium 33mg, Phosphorus 26mg, Potassium 67mg

Tips:

- This fritter recipe contains only 33mg of sodium when compared to donut shop apple fritters which approximately contains about 300mg sodium
- If desired, Splenda granular sugar can serve as a substitute for sugar

Gingerbread Muffins

Suitable For: CKD non-dialysis, dialysis, and diabetes

Preparation Time: 10 minutes; **Cooking Time:** 25 minutes; **Servings:** 12; **Serving Size:** 1 muffin

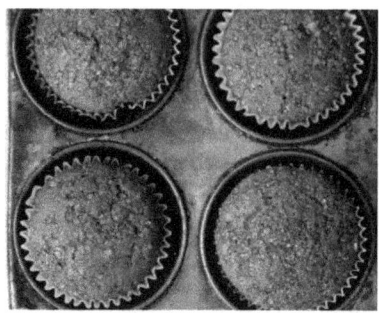

Ingredients:

- 2 large eggs
- ¾ cup of low-fat milk
- 6 tablespoons of canola oil
- ½ cup of brown sugar
- 4 tablespoons of dark corn syrup
- 2 cups of all-purpose flour
- 1 tablespoon of baking powder
- 4 teaspoons of ground ginger
- 1½ teaspoons of ground cinnamon

Directions:

1. Preheat oven to 400°, and grease a 12-cup muffin pan
2. Slightly beat the eggs in a medium-sized bowl. Also add in the milk, oil, brown sugar, corn syrup and beat
3. Using a large bowl, add in and stir the flour, baking powder, ginger, and cinnamon. Make a deep hole in the middle and add in the liquid

ingredients from step 2. Gently stir until contents are combined. Don't over mix
4. Scoop batter with a spoon and place it into the muffin pan. Place the muffin pan in the preheated oven and bake for about 20 minutes until it becomes firm to touch and turns golden brown
5. Remove the muffin pan from the oven and allow to cool for 5 minutes, then serve warm

Nutrients Per Serving: Calories 216, Protein 4g, Carbohydrates 32g, Fat 8g, Cholesterol 32mg, Sodium 154mg, Potassium 80mg, Phosphorus 81mg

Tips:

- Baking powder is contained in muffins and contributes to phosphorus content. Discuss with your dietitian if phosphate binder should be taken when having muffins

French Toast and Cream Cheese with Applesauce

Suitable For: CKD non-dialysis, dialysis, and diabetes

Preparation Time: 10 minutes; **Cooking Time:** 15 minutes; **Servings:** 1; **Serving Size:** 1

Ingredients:

- 2 slices of whole wheat bread
- 4 tablespoons of egg whites
- 1-ounce of cream cheese
- 2 tablespoons of unsweetened applesauce
- Cinnamon to taste

Directions:

1. Preheat a non-stick skillet over medium-high heat
2. Add two tablespoons of egg white on one side of a slice of bread and place in skillet
3. Add the cream cheese and applesauce to the bread. Sprinkle with cinnamon
4. Repeat step 2 using the other slice of bread, then place it above the slice in the pan with the egg side up
5. When the bottom of the first slice of bread turns brown, flip it to the other side and brown
6. Remove and place in a plate to serve and top with your preferred syrup

Nutrients Per Serving: Calories 276, Protein 16g, Carbohydrates 26g, Fat 12g, Cholesterol 33mg, Sodium

466mg, Potassium 314mg, Phosphorus 158mg, Fiber 5.4g

Tips:

- 66 mg of phosphorus is contained in one egg yolk. It is recommended that you use just the egg white so that you can use the whole wheat bread to increase fiber while keeping phosphorus low.

Spaghetti-Basil Frittata

Suitable For: CKD non-dialysis, dialysis, and diabetes

Preparation Time: 10 minutes; **Cooking Time:** 25 minutes; **Servings:** 4; **Serving Size:** 1 wedge

Ingredients:

- ⅓ cup of green onion
- 2 tablespoons of fresh basil
- 2 teaspoons of olive oil
- 2½ cups of whole wheat spaghetti, cooked
- ⅓ cup of low-fat milk
- 4 large eggs
- 2 large egg white
- ¼ teaspoon of black pepper
- 2 ounces of mozzarella cheese

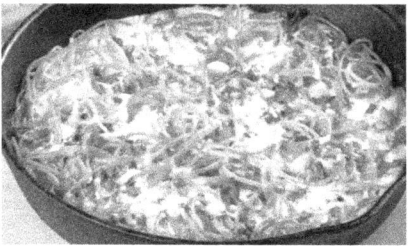

Directions:

1. Chop the green onion and basil, then set aside
2. Use two teaspoons of olive oil to grease a medium non-skillet
3. Evenly spread the cooked spaghetti in the skillet and cook for 2 minutes over medium heat
4. In a bowl, whisk the milk, eggs, egg white, and black pepper, then pour gently over the pasta. Sprinkle the frittata with the green onions, basil, and cheese, then cover and cook for about 8 minutes until it is set
5. Cut the frittata into four and serve

Nutrients Per Serving: Calories 271, Protein 17g, Carbohydrates 26g, Fat 11g, Cholesterol 196mg, Sodium 208mg, Potassium 212mg, Phosphorus 279mg, Fiber 3.1g

Tips:

- If preferred, you can substitute whole-wheat spaghetti for refined spaghetti

Berry Chia Pudding

Suitable For: CKD non-dialysis, dialysis, and diabetes

Preparation Time: 15 minutes; **Cooking Time:** 0 minutes; **Servings:** 4; **Serving Size:** ½ cup with berries

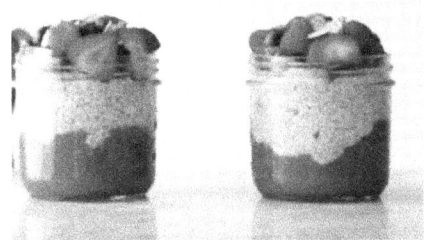

Ingredients:

- 2 cups of vanilla sweetened almond milk
- ½ cup of chia seeds
- ¼ cup of sweetened coconut, shredded
- ¼ cup of fresh blueberries
- 4 large strawberries

Directions:

1. Together in a blender, blend the chia seeds and almond milk.
2. Pour the mixture into four clear dessert dishes. Stir to distribute the chia seeds.
3. Refrigerate for about an hour in the refrigerator or ½ an hour in the freezer.
4. Before serving, use one tablespoon of the shredded coconut, one large strawberry and one tablespoon of blueberries to top the serving

Nutrients Per Serving: Calories 184, Protein 4g, Carbohydrates 22g, Fat 9g, Sodium 94mg, Potassium 199mg, Phosphorus 200mg, Fiber 8g

Asparagus and Cheese Crepe Rolls

Suitable For: CKD non-dialysis, dialysis, and diabetes

Preparation Time: 10 minutes; **Cooking Time:** 35 minutes; **Servings:** 4; **Serving Size:** 1

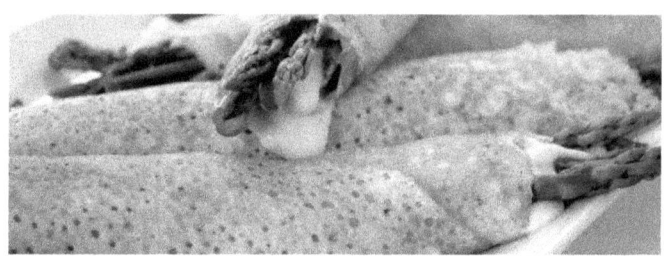

Ingredients:

- 12 asparagus spears
- 4 ounces of cream cheese
- 1 bundle parsley
- 1 teaspoon of lemon juice
- ½ teaspoon of black pepper
- ⅓ cup of all-purpose flour
- ½ cup of water
- ¼ cup of cream
- 1 egg
- 2 egg white
- 4 tablespoons of unsalted butter

Directions:

1. Steam the asparagus for about 6 to 8 minutes

2. Puree the cream cheese to make a green cream sauce by using the parsley, lemon juice, and pepper, then set aside
3. Mix the flour, water, egg, egg white and two tablespoons of melted butter to make the crepes, then whisk for a smooth batter
4. Melt ½ tablespoon of butter in a crepe or sauté pan, add ⅓ cup of crepe batter and then turn the pan for batter to spread. Cook until both sides of the batter become brown. Remove and place on a plate
5. Repeat to make four crepes altogether using the remaining butter and batter
5. Use the cream cheese filling to spread over the crepes, use the steamed asparagus to distribute evenly at each crepe's end, then roll up into rolls
6. Wrap the rolled crepe in a foil, and allow it cool for 1 hour in the refrigerator, then serve

Nutrients Per Serving: Calories 305, Protein 10g, Carbohydrates 16g, Fat 24g, Cholesterol 114mg, Sodium 247mg, Potassium 357mg, Phosphorus 142mg, Fiber 2.9g

Tips:

- Fill the crepe with shrimp rather than asparagus if you want a higher protein entrée. To do this, simply peel the shrimp, sauté in olive oil, allow it to cool down, then curl it up in the crepes

Breakfast Casserole

Suitable For: CKD non-dialysis, dialysis, and diabetes

Preparation Time: 10 minutes; **Cooking Time:** 55 minutes; **Servings:** 4; **Serving Size:** one 3 x 3-inch

Ingredients:

- 8 ounces of fat pork sausage
- 8 ounces of cream cheese
- 1 cup of low-fat milk
- 4 slices of cubed or broken white bread
- 5 large eggs
- ½ teaspoon of dry mustard
- ½ teaspoon of dried onion flakes

Directions:

1. Preheat the oven to about 325 F°
2. Crumble sausage and cook in a medium-size skillet, then set aside
3. Mix the remaining ingredients in a blender, excluding the bread
4. Add the cooked sausage to the mixture

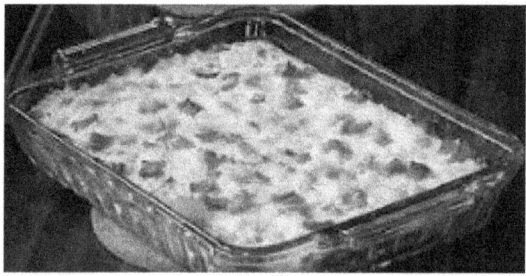

5. Place the pieces of bread into a greased 9x9 casserole dish, then pour the sausage mixture over bread
6. Bake for 55 minutes or until it is ready
7. Allow casserole to cool for about 10 minutes before cutting into serving size.

Nutrients Per Serving: Calories 224, Protein 11g, Carbohydrates 9g, Fat 16g, Cholesterol 149mg, Sodium 356mg, Potassium 201mg, Phosphorus 159mg, Fiber 0.4g

Grilled Corn and Cheesecakes (Arepas)

Suitable For: CKD non-dialysis, dialysis, and diabetes

Preparation Time: 10 minutes; **Cooking Time:** 20 minutes; **Servings:** 4; **Serving Size:** 1 corncake

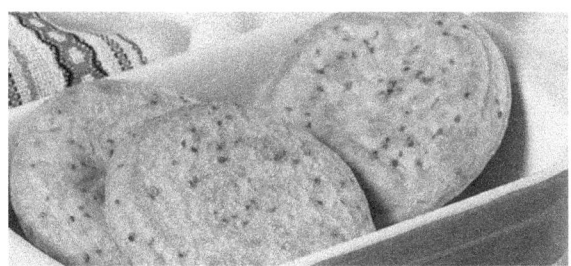

Ingredients:

- ⅔ cup of white cornflour
- 4 ounces of costeño cheese

- ½ teaspoon of anise
- 1 cup of hot water
- 1 teaspoon of unsalted butter

Directions:

1. Place cornflour in a bowl, grate the cheese, then add to the cornflour. Also, add the anise to the cornflour
2. Pour the hot water and mix using a spatula
3. Allow to rest for about 10 minutes then knead for about 2 to 3 minutes
4. Make a circle of 4 (ideally, about 4-inch wide and ½ -inch thick) to form the corn cakes
5. Use butter to grease a skillet, then place each corn cake to cook until slightly browned

Nutrients Per Serving: Calories 285, Protein 9g, Carbohydrates 40g, Fat 11g, Cholesterol 31mg, Sodium 409mg, Potassium 198mg, Phosphorus 344mg, Fiber 3.7g

Tips:

- Arepa flour is used, especially for making arepas. If unavailable, you can substitute for maza cornflour
- Although costeño cheese is a hard and salty cheese, you can substitute with cotija or Parmesan cheese

German Pancakes

Suitable For: CKD non-dialysis, dialysis, and diabetes

Preparation Time: 15 minutes; **Cooking Time:** 40 minutes; **Servings:** 10; **Serving Size:** 2 pancakes

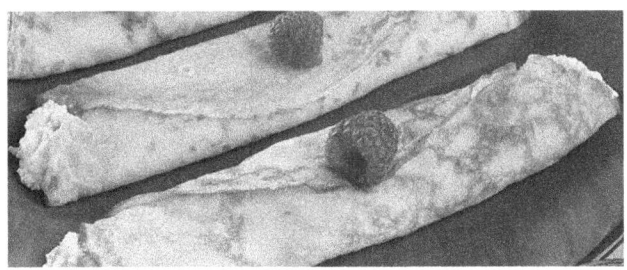

Ingredients:

- ⅔ cup of all-purpose flour
- 2 tablespoons of sugar
- 4 large eggs
- 1 cup of low-fat milk
- ¼ teaspoon of vanilla extract

Directions:

1. Mix the flour and sugar in a medium-size bowl, then add the eggs and blend properly using a whisk
2. Pour in the milk and vanilla extract, then beat continuously until it is smooth
3. Add three tablespoons of the batter into a heated 8 or 10-inch non-stick skillet that is sprayed with non-stick cooking spray.

4. Quickly tilt the pan to spread the batter, then cook until the pancake turns brown on the underside (edges will begin to dry at about 45 seconds). Flip the pancake and cook until the other side turns brown. Continue the process until all the batter has been used.
5. Roll or fold the pancakes, serving with spreads of fruit, syrup, or jam.

Nutrients Per Serving: Calories 74, Protein 4g, Carbohydrates 10g, Fat 2g, Cholesterol 76mg, Sodium 39mg, Potassium 73mg, Phosphorus 72mg, Fiber 0.2g

Tips:

- Use fruit spread or syrup that is sugar-free as a topping if you have diabetes

Homemade Turkey Sausage

Suitable For: CKD non-dialysis, dialysis, and diabetes

Preparation Time: 10 minutes; **Cooking Time:** 10 minutes; **Servings:** 12; **Serving Size:** 1 patty

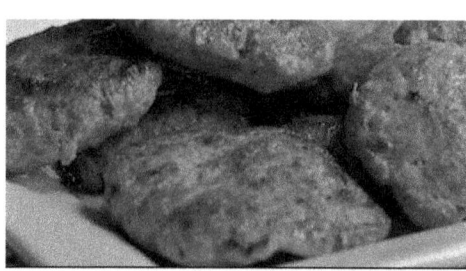

Ingredients:

- 1 teaspoon of fennel seed
- 1 pound of ground turkey

- ⅛ teaspoon of garlic powder
- ⅛ teaspoon of onion powder
- ¼ teaspoon of salt (or exclude to reduce sodium)

Directions:

1. Crush the fennel seed
2. Altogether, mix the turkey, crushed fennel seed, garlic powder, onion powder, and salt in a bowl, then cover and refrigerate overnight
3. Make ball portions of the seasoned turkey with your hand, and flatten into patties to cook
4. Use a non-stick skillet to cook over medium heat until both sides are browned

Nutrients Per Serving: Calories 55, Protein 7g, Fat 3g, Cholesterol 24mg, Carbohydrates 0g, Sodium 70mg, Potassium 106mg, Phosphorus 75mg, Fiber 0g

Tips:

- Refrigerate extra patties for later use. Make sure a double layer of waxed paper or wrap is placed between servings, this will allow for easy separation of patties

Homemade Belgian Waffles

Suitable For: CKD non-dialysis, dialysis, and diabetes

Preparation Time: 15 minutes; **Cooking Time:** 20 minutes; **Servings:** 6; **Serving Size:** 1 large waffle

Ingredients:

- 2 large eggs
- 2 cups of cake flour
- ¾ cup of low-fat milk
- ¾ teaspoon of baking soda
- ¾ cup of sour cream
- 2 tablespoons of granulated sugar
- 2 teaspoons of vanilla extract
- 4 tablespoons of unsalted butter
- 6 tablespoons of powdered sugar

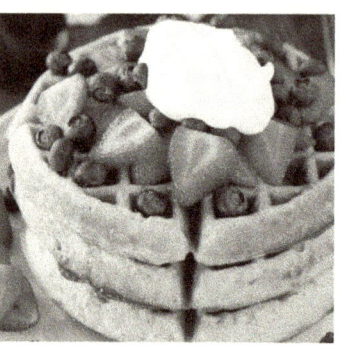

Directions:

1. Heat-up a waffle iron
2. Mix the cake flour and baking soda in a mixing bowl and set aside.
3. Separate the egg yolk and egg white, then whisk the egg yolk, milk, sour cream, and vanilla extract all together

4. Dissolve the butter by melting and then mix into the mixture from step 3.
5. Beat the egg white in another bowl using a hand mixer until soft peaks are formed (about 2 minutes). Add the granulated sugar to the egg white, then beat with the hand-mixer until stiff peaks are formed (about 3-4 extra minutes)
6. Whisk the mixture from step 4 into the flour mixture from step 2, and then gently mix with the beaten egg white from step 5 until the mixture is smooth
7. Pour about ½ cup of the batter to the heated waffle iron, close and then cook for 3 minutes
8. Serve waffles alongside the powdered sugar. If you choose to, include toppings such as fresh berries (strawberries, blueberries or raspberries), jam or syrup

Nutrients Per Serving: Calories 367, Protein 8g, Carbohydrates 50g, Fat 15g, Cholesterol 98mg, Sodium 204mg, Potassium 151mg, Phosphorus 121mg, Fiber 1g

Tips:

- You can substitute the powdered sugar for maple syrup, and if used, ¼ cup contains 54g of carbohydrate and 170mg of potassium. On the other hand, some imitation pancake or light syrup may contain phosphorus additives; if you

want to use such, ensure you read the ingredient label to avoid these additives
- Strawberries, raspberries, or blueberries may also be used as toppings for these waffles. ½ cup of berries would add about 5-10g of carbohydrate and 55-110mg of potassium, which depends on the type of fruit used
- If you have diabetes and want to reduce the carbohydrate level, change the serving size to ½ waffle, topped with berries and whipped cream. This would reduce the amount of carbohydrate to around 30-35g

Chapter 4

Soups and Stew

Maryland Cream of Crab Soup

Suitable For: CKD non-dialysis, dialysis, and diabetes

Preparation Time: 10 minutes; **Cooking Time:** 30 minutes; **Servings:** 7; **Serving Size:** 1 cup

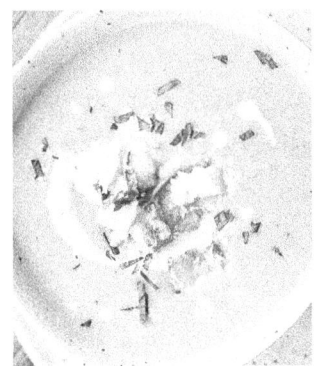

Ingredients:

- 1 tablespoon of unsalted butter
- 1 cup of onion
- ½ pound of fresh lump crab meat
- 4 cups of low-sodium chicken broth
- 1 cup of liquid nondairy creamer
- 2 tablespoons of cornstarch
- ⅛ teaspoon of dill weed

- ⅛ teaspoon of Old Bay Seasoning
- ⅛ teaspoon of black pepper

Directions:

1. Using a large pot, melt the butter over medium heat
2. Chop the onion and add it to the pot. Cook, and stir until the onion is soft and transparent
3. Add the crab meat and cook for 2 to 3 minutes, stirring regularly
4. Add in the chicken broth, bringing the mixture to a boil. Reduce the heat to low
5. Use a small bowl to combine the nondairy creamer and cornstarch, then whisk until it becomes smooth. Add the mixture to the soup from step 4 and slightly increase the heat. Stir constantly until it thickens
6. Add in the dill weed, Old Bay seasoning, and pepper to the soup.

Nutrients Per Serving: Calories 142, Protein 12g, Carbohydrates 10g, Fat 6g, Cholesterol 29mg, Sodium 295mg, Potassium 244mg, Phosphorus 100mg, Fiber 0.3g

Tips:

- Fresh Maryland lump crabmeat is recommended as the best; however, you can use other varieties if unavailable
- Old Bay Seasoning is a popular seasoning which has about 160mg of sodium for a ¼ teaspoon. Substitute for other low-sodium seasonings if unavailable
- Get a low-sodium broth that has less than 250mg sodium per cup, and avoid low-sodium broth with potassium chloride –because it contains high potassium levels.

Rotisserie Chicken Noodle Soup

Suitable For: CKD non-dialysis, dialysis, and diabetes

Preparation Time: 10 minutes; **Cooking Time:** 25 minutes; **Servings:** 10; **Serving Size:** 1¼ cups

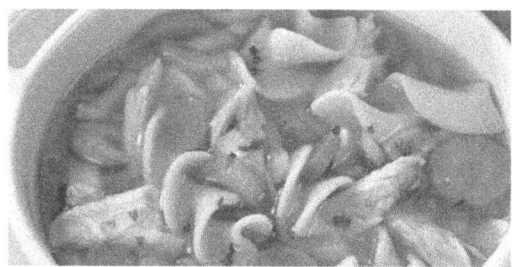

Ingredients:

- 1 prepared rotisserie chicken
- 8 cups of low-sodium chicken broth
- ½ cup of onion
- 1 cup of celery
- 1 cup of carrots
- 6 ounces of uncooked wide noodles
- 3 tablespoons of fresh parsley

Directions:

1. Remove the chicken from the bones, chop into pieces of bite-sized, and measure 4 cups for the soup
2. Use a large stockpot and pour in the chicken broth, then bring to a boil
3. Chop the onion, and slice the celery and carrots
4. Add the chicken, vegetables, and the noodles to the stockpot, and bring to a boil. Cook for approximately 15 minutes or until the noodles are done
5. Garnish with chopped parsley

Nutrients Per Serving: Calories 185, Protein 21g, Carbohydrates 14g, Fat 5g, Cholesterol 63mg, Sodium 361mg, Potassium 294mg, Phosphorus 161mg, Fiber 1.4g

Tips:

- Low-sodium broth is made up of about 140mg sodium or less per cup. You can use Campbell's low-sodium broth, Nature's Choice low-sodium broth, or Health Valley low-sodium broth. Try avoiding low-sodium broth that has potassium chloride in its ingredient label— it has high potassium content

Irish Lamb Stew

Suitable For: CKD non-dialysis, dialysis, and diabetes

Preparation Time: 10 minutes; **Cooking Time:** 1 hr 35 minutes; **Servings:** 6; **Serving Size:** 1 cup

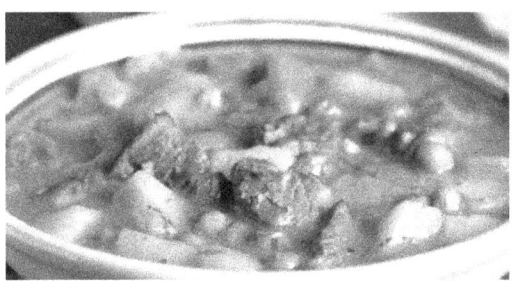

Ingredients:

- 1½ pounds of lamb shoulder, boneless
- ½ teaspoon of salt (or exclude to reduce sodium)
- ½ teaspoon of black pepper
- 1 tablespoon of olive oil

- 1 medium-sized onion
- ¼ cup of all-purpose flour
- 3 garlic cloves
- 1 teaspoon of dried thyme
- ½ cup of tomato sauce
- 1 cup of stout beer
- 2 cups of low-sodium beef broth
- 2 medium-sized carrots
- 2 medium-sized parsnips
- 1 cup of frozen green peas

Directions:

1. Cut lamb into 1 ½ chunk and dice the onion and garlic
2. Place the pieces of lamb on a plate, then sprinkle using salt and pepper
3. Place flour in a zip-top bag, add the lamb, then shake until meat is evenly coated
4. Over medium heat in a Dutch oven or a large stockpot, heat the one tablespoon of olive oil, add the lamb, then cook until it is browned evenly. Take it off from the pot and put aside
5. To the same pot, add the onion and fry until it is translucent. Add the diced garlic, stir for a minute, then add ½ cup of beef broth and stir to deglaze the pot.
6. Add the lamb, the remaining beef broth, tomato sauce, beer, and thyme to the pot. Reduce to low heat and cook. Simmer for 1 hour.

7. Cut into 1-inch pieces, the carrots, and parsnips, stir into the stew, then simmer for another 30 minutes.
8. Add green peas then cook for about 5 to 10 minutes.

Nutrients Per Serving: Calories 283, Protein 27g, Carbohydrates 19g, Fat 11g, Cholesterol 80mg, Sodium 325mg, Potassium 527mg, Phosphorus 300mg Fiber 3.4g

Tips:

- If you cannot get boneless lamb shoulder, then get 2½ pounds of lamb shoulder, chopped and trimmed of fat and bones
- If you have CKD non-dialysis and want to lower your protein diet further, then reduce lamb to ¾ pounds, this would cut down protein diet to 15g. Nonetheless, consult with your dietitian on the amount that is best for your diet.

Creamy Broccoli Soup

Suitable For: CKD non-dialysis, dialysis, and diabetes

Preparation Time: 10 minutes; **Cooking Time:** 20 minutes; **Servings:** 5; **Serving Size:** 1 cup

Ingredients:

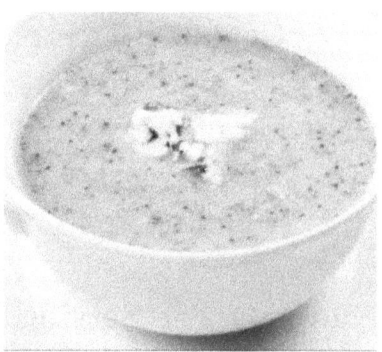

- 2 cups of low-sodium vegetable broth
- 3 cups of broccoli florets
- 8 ounces of undrained silken tofu
- 3 tablespoons of cornstarch
- 3 tablespoons of nutritional yeast
- 1 teaspoon of onion powder
- 1 teaspoon of garlic powder
- ¼ teaspoon of black pepper
- ⅛ teaspoon of red pepper flakes

Directions:

1. Boil the broccoli florets and tofu (including the liquid) in the vegetable broth using a large pot, and allow to cook until it is tender. Put aside to cool
2. Pour the cooled contents into a large mixing bowl and use an immersion blender to blend until it becomes smooth.
3. Mix 1 ½ cups of the soup with the cornstarch in a small bowl, then whisk until it becomes smooth.
4. Pour the soup back into the pot, add the mixed cornstarch and boil. Add the nutritional yeast and all other spices, then stir until well combined.

Nutrients Per Serving: Calories 65, Protein 4g, Carbohydrates 10g, Fat 1g, Sodium 71mg, Potassium 289mg, Phosphorus 90mg, Fiber 1.7g

Tips:

- This soup is a great choice for people that have difficulty in swallowing or chewing
- You can substitute vegetable broth for low-sodium chicken broth if desired

Southwestern Posole

Suitable For: CKD non-dialysis, dialysis, and diabetes

Preparation Time: 10 minutes; Cooking Time: 50 minutes; Servings: 6; Serving Size: 1½ cups

Ingredients:

- 1 tablespoon of olive oil
- 1 pound of pork loin
- ½ cup of onion
- 1 garlic clove
- 28 ounces canned of white hominy
- 4 ounces of canned diced green chiles
- 4 cups of low-sodium chicken broth

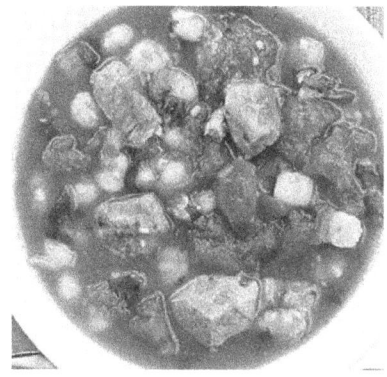

- ¼ teaspoon of black pepper

Directions:

1. Cut the pork into pieces of 1-inch, then chop the onion and the garlic. Drain and rinse the hominy
2. Using a skillet, heat oil over medium heat and brown the pieces of pork for about 3 to 4 minutes
3. Add the onion and garlic to the skillet, then sauté until the onion is tender
4. Add the remaining ingredients and simmer for about 30 to 45 minutes or until the meat becomes tender and the flavors are mixed
5. Add water if additional liquid is required

Nutrients Per Serving: Calories 286, Protein 26g, Carbohydrates 15g, Fat 13g, Cholesterol 63mg, Sodium 399mg, Potassium 346mg, Phosphorus 182mg, Fiber 3.4g

Tips:

- You can substitute green chiles for 1 to 2 tablespoons of red chili powder
- If you have CKD non-dialysis and want to lower your protein diet further, then reduce the pork in this recipe. Nonetheless, consult with your dietitian on the amount that is best for your diet.

Red Lentil Dahl

Suitable For: CKD non-dialysis, dialysis, and diabetes

Preparation Time: 10 minutes; **Cooking Time:** 30 minutes; **Servings:** 4; **Serving Size:** ¼ of recipe

Ingredients:

- 1 cup of red lentils
- 1 tablespoon of canola oil
- ½ teaspoon of cumin seeds

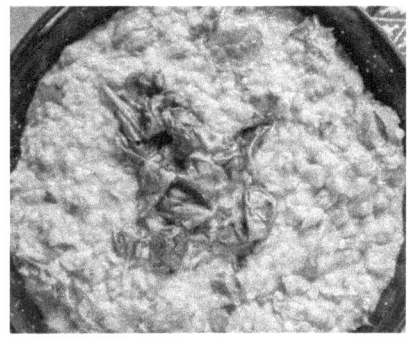

- 1 (2-inch of cinnamon stick)
- 1 cup of diced yellow onion
- 1 green minced chili pepper
- 4 minced garlic cloves
- 1 tablespoon of minced ginger root
- ½ teaspoon of ground turmeric
- ½ teaspoon ground cardamom
- ½ teaspoon of paprika
- ¼ teaspoon of kosher salt (or exclude to reduce sodium)
- 1 medium-sized diced tomato
- 1½ Juice of lemon
- Chopped cilantro leaves

Directions:

To prepare the lentils:

1. In a bowl of water, soak the lentils for about 12 hours or more
2. Rinse the lentils to get rid of the soaked water
3. Using a medium-sized saucepan, add in the rinsed lentils along with 3 cups of water (at room temperature), then bring to a boil over medium heat and cook for 20 minutes

To prepare the seasonings:

1. Using a medium-sized skillet, heat the canola oil over medium heat, then add the cumin seeds, cinnamon stick and cook for about 1 minute 30 seconds until fragrant
2. Add in the onion, pepper, ginger, garlic and cook for about 6 minutes until the onions become translucent
3. Add in the turmeric, paprika, cardamom, salt, and tomato. Cook for about 3 minutes and discard the cinnamon stick
4. Once the lentils are ready, drain any extra water, and stir in the spiced onion mixture (from step 2and 3). Also, stir in the lemon juice
5. Garnish lentil soup with cilantro and serve with basmati rice

Nutrients Per Serving: Calories 230, Sodium 105 mg, Phosphorus 169mg, Potassium 32mg, Fiber 7g, Protein 13g, Carbohydrates 37g

Tips:
- Soaking the lentils for about 12 hours or more drastically reduces potassium levels by 93%

Shrimp and Crab Gumbo

Suitable For: CKD non-dialysis, dialysis, and diabetes

Preparation Time: 10 minutes; **Cooking Time:** 25 minutes; **Servings:** 6; **Serving Size:** 1 cup

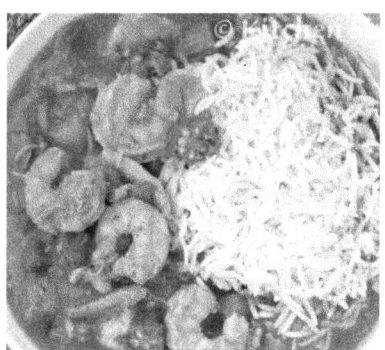

Ingredients:

- 1 cup of bell pepper
- 1½ cups of onion
- 1 garlic clove
- ¼ of cup celery leaves
- 1 cup of green onion tops

- ¼ cup of fresh parsley
- 4 tablespoons of canola oil
- 6 tablespoons of all-purpose white flour
- 3 cups of water
- 4 cups of low-sodium chicken broth
- 8 ounces of uncooked shrimp
- 6 ounces of crab meat
- ¼ teaspoon of black pepper
- 1 teaspoon of hot sauce
- 3 cups of cooked rice

Directions:

1. Chop the bell peppers, garlic, celery, onion, green onion tops, and parsley
2. To make a roux, use a large skillet and heat oil and flour over medium heat. Stir until flour is color pecan
3. Add in the bell peppers, onion, celery, garlic, and 1 cup of water. Cover and cook over low heat until the vegetables become tender
4. Over high heat, add in 2 cups of water and 4 cups of the low sodium chicken broth, then boil for about for 5 minutes
5. Over medium heat, add in the shrimp and crab meat, then boil for additional 10 minutes
6. Add in the green onion tops and parsley, then reduce the heat to low heat. Simmer for 5 minutes
7. Add pepper and hot sauce to season, then serve with rice

Nutrients Per Serving: Calories 327, Fat 11g, Protein 22g, Sodium 328mg, Fiber 1.4g, Phosphorus 221mg, Potassium 368 mg, Cholesterol 86 mg, Carbohydrates 33g,

Tips:

- Roux comes in different flavors, which depends on how long the flour is cooked. Cook until the roux becomes coffee color, for a deeper flavor
- Either fresh, canned or frozen lump crabmeat can be used

Ground Beef Soup

Suitable For: CKD non-dialysis, dialysis, and diabetes

Preparation Time: 15 minutes; **Cooking Time:** 35 minutes; **Servings:** 6; **Serving Size:** 1¼ cups

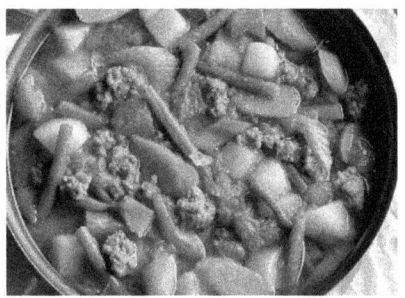

Ingredients:

- 1 pound of lean ground beef

- ½ cup of onion
- 2 teaspoons of Mrs. Dash lemon pepper
- 1 teaspoon of kitchen Bouquet seasoning and browning sauce
- 1 cup of reduced-sodium beef broth
- 2 cups of water
- ⅓ cup of uncooked brown rice
- 3 cups of frozen mixed vegetables (green beans, corn, peas, and carrots)
- 1 tablespoon of sour cream

Directions:

1. Slice the onion, brown the ground beef with the onion in a large saucepan, then drain fat
2. Add in the seasoning and browning sauce, beef broth, water, rice, and the mixed vegetables
3. Bring to a boil over high heat. Then reduce heat to medium-low, cover and cook for about 30 minutes
4. Take off from heat, and stir in the sour cream

Nutrients Per Serving: Calories 222, Protein 20g, Fat 8g, Cholesterol 52mg, Sodium 170mg, Potassium 448mg, Fiber 4.3g, Phosphorus 210mg, Carbohydrates 204g,

Tips:

- Use a reduced-sodium beef broth with 500 mg of sodium or less per 1 cup serving and avoid using low-sodium beef broth with potassium chloride

content – this is because potassium chloride low-sodium beef broth has high potassium levels. You can prepare your own homemade low-sodium broth to use in this recipe
- Other vegetable mixture you can use as a substitute are cauliflower, carrots and snow peas — this lowers the phosphorus level to 190 mg per serving

Yucatan Chicken Lime Soup

Suitable For: CKD non-dialysis, dialysis, and diabetes

Preparation Time: 15 minutes; **Cooking Time:** 30 minutes; **Servings:** 4; **Serving Size:** 1½ cups

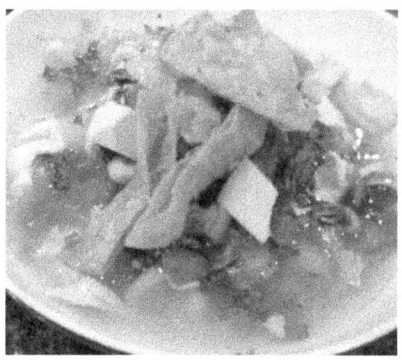

Ingredients:

- ½ cup of onion
- 8 cloves of garlic
- 2 Serrano chili peppers

- 1 medium-sized tomato
- 1½ cups of uncooked chicken breast
- 2 (6-inch) corn tortillas
- Non-stick cooking spray
- 1 tablespoon of olive oil
- 4 cups of low-sodium chicken broth
- ¼ of teaspoon salt (or exclude to reduce sodium)
- 1 bay leaf
- ¼ cup of lime juice
- ¼ cup of fresh cilantro
- ½ teaspoon of black pepper

Directions:

1. Preheat oven to 400º F
2. Chop the onion and cilantro, then mince the garlic cloves. Slice the chili peppers, and cut the tomato into half and remove its skin and seeds. Shred the chicken
3. Cut into strips, the tortillas, and arrange it on a baking sheet. Spray with cooking spray, then bake for about 3 minutes or until it becomes slightly toasted. Take off from oven, placing it on a plate to cool
4. In a large saucepan, heat the oil over medium heat. Add the onion, garlic, and chili peppers, then cook until the onions become translucent.
5. Add the tomato, broth, chicken breast, bay leaf, and salt. Simmer for about 8 to 10 minutes

6. Add the lime juice and the fresh cilantro, then season using the black pepper. Taste, and add extra juice if desired
7. Serve and top with strips of tortilla

Nutrients Per Serving: Calories 214, Protein 20g, Carbohydrates 12g, Fat 10g, Cholesterol 32mg, Sodium 246mg, Potassium 355mg, Phosphorus 176mg, Fiber 1.6g

Tips:
- Homemade chicken stock has about 30 to 60mg sodium per cup, without adding salt or bouillon. Low-sodium or no-salt-added broth has less than 140mg sodium of per cup, while reduced-sodium broth has about 450 to 600mg sodium per cup
- If you wish to use reduced-sodium broth for this recipe, then decrease the broth amount to 2 cups, omit the ¼ teaspoon of salt and add 2 cups of water to lower the sodium level

Italian Wedding Soup

Suitable For: CKD non-dialysis, dialysis, and diabetes

Preparation Time: 15 minutes; **Cooking Time:** 30 minutes; **Servings:** 10; **Serving Size:** 1½ cups

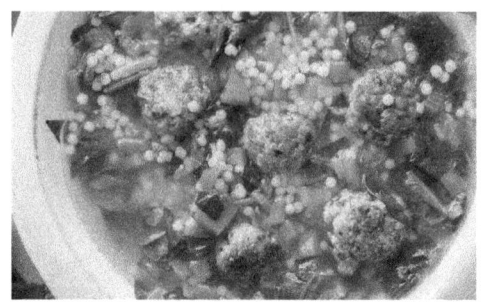

Ingredients:

- 1 pound of extra-lean ground beef
- 2 eggs, beaten
- ¼ cup of dried bread crumbs
- 2 tablespoons of grated parmesan cheese
- 1 teaspoon of dried basil
- 3 tablespoons of onion
- 2½ quarts of low-sodium chicken broth
- 1 cup of fresh spinach leaves
- 1 cup of uncooked acini de pepe pasta
- ¾ cup of carrots
- 2 cups of cooked chicken

Directions:

1. Cut the spinach leaves, dice the carrots and chicken, and mince the onions
2. Add in a bowl the beef, bread crumbs, beaten eggs, cheese, basil, and onion, then mix thoroughly

3. Roll the mixed beef into a ½ -inch diameter log, cut into 80 pieces, roll into tiny meatballs, then put aside
4. Heat the chicken broth to boil using a large stockpot.
5. Add in the spinach, pasta, carrots, and meatballs, and stir. Reduce the heat to medium
6. Cook at a slow boil for about 10 minutes (stirring frequently) or until the pasta is "al dente" and meatballs are no longer pink on the inside
7. Pour in the diced chicken and allow the chicken to heat thoroughly.
8. Serve hot

Nutrients Per Serving: Calories 165, Protein 21g, Carbohydrates 11g, Fat 6g, Cholesterol 73mg, Sodium 276mg, Potassium 360mg, Phosphorus 176mg, Fiber 1.0g

Tips:

- Use low-sodium broth that has no potassium chloride. If unavailable, use reduced-sodium broth or better still, prepare a homemade low-sodium broth

Beef and Barley Stew

Suitable For: CKD non-dialysis, dialysis, and diabetes

Preparation Time: 20 minutes; **Cooking Time:** 1 hr 35 minutes; **Servings:** 6; **Serving Size:** 1¼

Ingredients:

- 1 cup of uncooked pearl barley
- 1 pound of lean beef stew meat
- 2 tablespoons of all-purpose white flour
- ¼ teaspoon of black pepper
- ¼ teaspoon of salt (or exclude to reduce sodium)
- 2 tablespoons of canola oil
- ½ cup of onion
- 1 large stalk celery
- 1 garlic clove
- 2 medium-sized carrots
- 2 bay leaves
- 1 teaspoon of Mrs. Dash onion herb seasoning

Directions:

1. Place the barley in 2 cups of water and soak for an hour
2. Dice the onion and celery, mince the garlic clove, slice the carrots into ¼-inch thick, and cut the beef into cubes of 1½inch.
3. Place flour in a zip-top bag, add black pepper, and stew meat, then shake until the meat is evenly coated
4. Heat oil using a 4-quart pot and brown the stew meat. Take the stew meat off the pot
5. Sauté and stir in meat drippings the onion, celery, and garlic for 2 minutes, then add 2 quarts of water and boil
6. Return the meat to the pot, add salt and bay leaves, and reduce the heat to a simmer
7. Drain and rinse the barley, pour into the pot, cover, and then cook for 1 hour. Stirring every 15 minutes
8. After 1 hour, add carrots and Mrs. Dash seasoning. Simmer for about 30 minutes. Add extra water if necessary to prevent sticking

Nutrients Per Serving: Calories 246, Protein 22g, Carbohydrates 21g, Fat 8g, Cholesterol 51mg, Sodium 222mg, Potassium 369mg, Phosphorus 175mg, Fiber 6.3g

Tips:

- For a lower protein diet CKD non-dialysis, reduce the beef to 8 ounces per recipe. This will decrease the amount of protein to 14g per serving

Beef and Cabbage Borscht Soup

Suitable For: CKD non-dialysis, dialysis, and diabetes

Preparation Time: 15 minutes; **Cooking Time:** 2 hr; **Servings:** 12; **Serving Size:** 1¼ cup

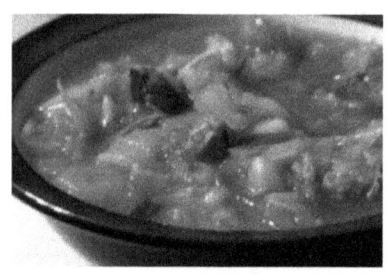

Ingredients:

- 2 pounds of beef blade steaks
- 6 cups of cold water
- 2 tablespoons of olive oil
- ½ cup of low-sodium tomato sauce
- 1 medium-sized cabbage
- 1 cup of onion
- 1 cup of carrots
- 1 cup of turnips
- ¾ teaspoon of salt (or exclude to reduce sodium)
- 1 teaspoon of pepper
- tablespoons of lemon juice
- 4 tablespoons of sugar

Directions:

1. Place the steak in a large pot, add water to completely cover the meat, cover, and bring to a boil. After the water begins to boil, reduce the heat to simmer, then cook until the meat becomes tender
2. Take the meat off the pot, shredding with a fork
3. Cut the cabbage into pieces of bite-size, dice onion, carrots, and turnips
4. With the meat broth still in the pot, add the olive oil, tomato sauce, cabbage, carrots, turnips, onion, and shredded meat
5. Add salt and pepper to season, then add the lemon juice and sugar
6. Allow to cook on low heat for about 1 to 1½hours until all the vegetables are well cooked.
7. Taste for seasoning, adding extra lemon, sugar or pepper if desired

Nutrients Per Serving: Calories 202, Protein 19g, Carbohydrates 9g, Fat 10g, Cholesterol 60mg, Sodium 242mg, Potassium 388mg, Phosphorus 160mg, Fiber 2.1g

Tips:

- Blade or cross-rib steak or roast may be used as a substitute
- Use light rye bread to serve with Cabbage Borscht

Seafood Corn Chowder Soup

Suitable For: CKD non-dialysis, dialysis, and diabetes

Preparation Time: 10 minutes; **Cooking Time:** 15 minutes; **Servings:** 10; **Serving Size:** 1 cup

Ingredients:

- 1 tablespoon of unsalted butter
- 1 cup of onion
- ⅓ cup of celery
- ½ cup of green bell pepper
- ½ cup of red bell pepper
- 1 tablespoon of all-purpose white flour
- 14 ounces of low-sodium chicken broth
- 2 cups of liquid non-dairy creamer
- 6 ounces of evaporated milk
- 10 ounces of surimi imitation crab chunks
- 2 cups of frozen corn kernels
- ½ teaspoon of black pepper
- ½ teaspoon of paprika

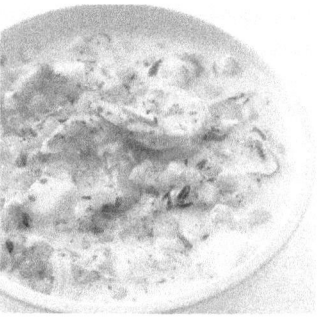

Directions:

1. Chop the onion, celery, and peppers
2. Melt the butter in a saucepan over medium heat, then cook the onion, celery, and peppers for about 5 minutes until it becomes tender

3. Pour in the flour, cook and stir continuously for about 2 minutes
4. Add in the chicken broth gradually, stir to blend and bring to a boil
5. Add in the non-dairy creamer, surimi, corn, evaporated milk, black pepper, and paprika
6. Heat and stir occasionally for about 5 minutes, then serve

Nutrients Per Serving: Calories 173, Fat 7g, Cholesterol 22mg, Sodium 160mg, Potassium 285mg, Carbohydrates 2g, Fiber 1.5g, Protein 8g, Phosphorus 181mg

Spring Vegetable Soup

Suitable For: CKD non-dialysis, dialysis, and diabetes

Preparation Time: 15 minutes; **Cooking Time:** 45 minutes; **Servings:** 5; **Serving Size:** 1 cup

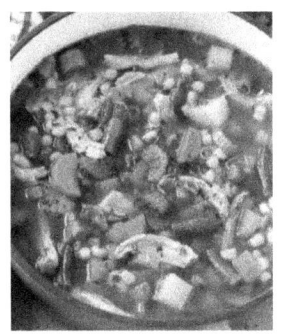

Ingredients:

- 1 cup of fresh green beans
- ¾ cup of celery
- ½ cup of onion
- ½ cup of carrots
- ½ cup of mushrooms
- 1 medium-sized Roma tomato
- 2 tablespoons of olive oil
- ½ cup of frozen corn
- 4 cups of low-sodium vegetable broth
- 1 teaspoon of dried oregano leaves
- 1 teaspoon of garlic powder
- ¼ teaspoon of salt (or exclude to reduce sodium)

Directions:

1. Take off the tips and strings from the green beans and cut into pieces (2-inch). Dice the celery, carrots, onion, mushrooms and tomato
2. Heat the olive oil in a large pot, and sauté only the celery and onion until it becomes tender
3. Add the other ingredients and bring to a boil. Reduce heat to simmer for about 45 to 60 minutes

Nutrients Per Serving: Calories 114, Protein 2g, Carbohydrates 13g, Fat 6g, Sodium 262mg, Potassium 400mg, Phosphorus 108mg, Fiber 3.4g

Chili Con Carne

Suitable For: CKD non-dialysis, dialysis, and diabetes

Preparation Time: 10 minutes; **Cooking Time:** 30 minutes; **Servings:** 8; **Serving Size:** 1 cup

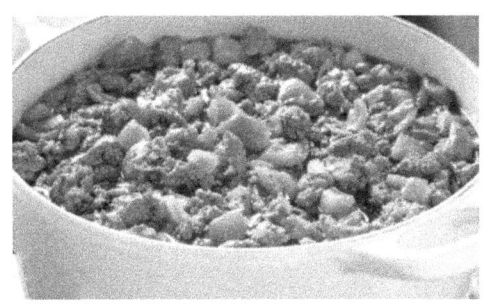

Ingredients:

- ½ cup of onion
- 1 stalk of celery
- ½ cup of green bell pepper
- 1½ pounds of lean ground beef
- 16 ounces of low-sodium stewed tomatoes
- 1 tablespoon of canola oil
- 2 tablespoons of chili powder
- 1½ cup of water

Directions:

1. Slice onion, celery and bell pepper

2. Use large skillet and heat over medium heat. Add oil, sliced onion, celery, and bell pepper, and cook until it becomes tender, but not brown
3. Break ground beef into small pieced and cook until it becomes brown
4. Liquefy the tomatoes in a blender, then add to the ground beef. Also, add the chili powder and water, combine thoroughly, reduce heat to low and simmer until it is cooked
5. Serve with low sodium crackers or hot rice

Nutrients Per Serving: Calories 190, Protein 20g, Carbohydrates 5g, Fat 10g, Cholesterol 57mg, Sodium 116mg, Potassium 450mg, Phosphorus 180mg, Fiber 1.25g

Chapter 5

Snacks and Appetizers

Barbecue Meatballs

Suitable For: CKD non-dialysis, dialysis, and diabetes

Preparation Time: 15 minutes; **Cooking Time:** 20 minutes; **Servings:** 24; **Serving Size:** 2 meatballs

Ingredients:

- ½ cup of onion
- 3 pounds of ground beef
- 2 large eggs
- ½ cup of unenriched rice milk
- 1 cup of uncooked oatmeal
- 1 tablespoon of dried thyme
- 1 teaspoon of dried oregano
- ½ teaspoon of pepper
- 1 cup of low sodium barbecue sauce
- ⅓ cup of water

Directions:

1. Preheat oven to 375° F
2. Dice the onion and beat the eggs

3. Mix all the ingredients in a large bowl, except the barbecue sauce and water
4. Roll mixed ingredients into 1-inch balls and place them on a baking sheet
5. Bake for about 20 minutes or until the meatballs cook through
6. Use a crockpot or warming dish to mix the barbecue sauce and water over low heat. Stir in the meatballs and cook for additional 20 minutes. Cover until ready to serve

Nutrients Per Serving: Calories 176, Protein 11g, Carbohydrates 6g, Fat 12g, Cholesterol 55mg, Sodium 180mg, Potassium 208mg, Phosphorus 107mg, Fiber 0.5g

Hot Crab Dip

Suitable For: CKD non-dialysis, dialysis, and diabetes

Preparation Time: 10 minutes; **Cooking Time:** 15 minutes; **Servings:** 10; **Serving Size:** 3 tablespoons

Ingredients:

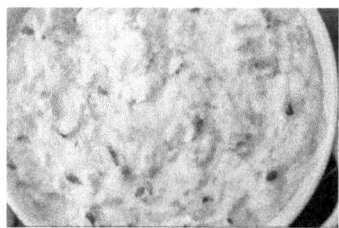

- 8 ounces of cream cheese
- 1 tablespoon of onion
- 1 teaspoon of lemon juice
- 2 teaspoons of Worcestershire sauce

- ⅛ teaspoon of black pepper
- ⅛ teaspoon of cayenne pepper
- 2 tablespoons of low-fat milk
- 6 ounces canned of crab meat

Directions:

1. Preheat oven to 375º F
2. Set out the cream cheese to soften, and mince the onion
3. Use a bowl and place the softened cream cheese
4. Add in and mix the onion, lemon juice, Worcestershire sauce, black pepper, and cayenne pepper. Stir in the milk
5. Stir in the crab meat until it blends in
6. Place the mixture on an oven-safe dish, then bake uncovered for about 15 minutes or until it becomes hot and bubbly

Nutrients Per Serving: Calories 96, Protein 8g, Carbohydrates 1g, Fat 8g, Cholesterol 42mg, Sodium 191mg, Potassium 92mg, Phosphorus 68mg, Fiber 0g

Tips:

- You can serve warm and with low-sodium crackers
- You can also try out this recipe with a freshly steamed crab meat rather than canned crab meat

Lemonade Chicken Wings

Suitable For: CKD non-dialysis, dialysis, and diabetes

Preparation Time: 10 minutes; **Cooking Time:** 35 minutes; **Servings:** 12; **Serving Size:** 2

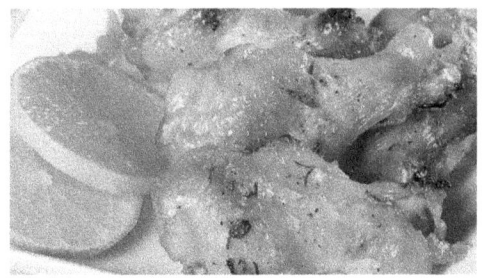

Ingredients:

- ¼ cup of onion
- 4 teaspoons of fresh rosemary
- ¼ cup of canola oil
- ¼ cup of unsalted butter
- 1 cup of lemonade
- 2 teaspoons of black pepper
- 24 chicken wing of drummettes

Directions:

1. Preheat oven to 400° F
2. Chop the onion and rosemary
3. Use a baking dish to place the chicken wings
4. Use a saucepan to add the remaining ingredients. Cook for about 3 minutes

5. Spread the mixed ingredients over the chicken, then bake for about 30 to 35 minutes or until it is set
6. Serve wings hot or place in a warming dish or crockpot until you are set to serve

Nutrients Per Serving: Calories 200, Protein 11g, Carbohydrates 3g, Fat 16g, Cholesterol 34mg, Sodium 67mg, Potassium 88mg, Phosphorus 62mg, Fiber 0.3g

Tips:

- If fresh wing drummettes are not available at the grocery, tell your butcher to cut whole chicken wings into the size of drummette
- If sugar-free lemonade is used, the carbohydrate level would be less than 1 gram. Check the lemonade label ingredients and avoid brands with phosphate additives
- Also, pieces of boneless chicken can be used

Tortilla Rollups

Suitable For: CKD non-dialysis, dialysis, and diabetes

Preparation Time: 15 minutes; **Cooking Time:** 0 minutes; **Servings:** 4; **Serving Size:** 3 pieces

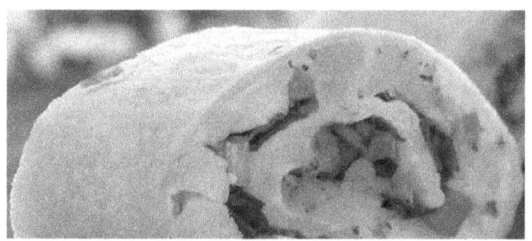

Ingredients:

- ½ cup of raw spinach leaves
- 2 tablespoons of onion
- 2 tablespoons of pimento
- 3 ounces of unprocessed and cooked turkey breast
- ½ cup of crushed pineapple
- ½ cup of whipped cream cheese
- 2 flour of burrito size tortillas
- 1 teaspoon of Mrs. Dash herb seasoning blend

Directions:

1. Chop the spinach, and dice the onion, pimento, and turkey breast. Also, drain the pineapple.
2. Spread the cream cheese over each tortilla, then sprinkle with Mrs. Dash seasoning
3. Use a bowl and mix in the remaining ingredients
4. Divide the mixed ingredients into two portions, place half on each tortilla then roll up
5. Trim the ends, slicing each roll in 6 pieces

Nutrients Per Serving: Calories 223, Protein 10g, Carbohydrates 21g, Fat 11g, Cholesterol 39mg, Sodium

298mg, Potassium 199mg, Phosphorus 126mg, Fiber 1.7g

Tips:

- Compare brands of tortilla and select the lowest in sodium

Cinnamon Yogurt Fruit Dip

Suitable For: CKD non-dialysis, dialysis, and diabetes

Preparation Time: 1 hr; **Cooking Time:** 0 minutes; **Servings:** 8; **Serving Size:** 2 spoons

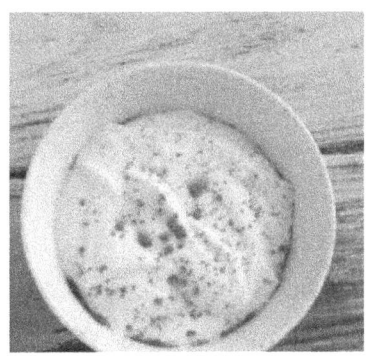

Ingredients:

- 4 ounces of light cream cheese
- 6 ounces of low-fat and Greek vanilla flavor yogurt
- ¼ cup of Polaner All Fruit and Strawberry Spreadable Fruit Fiber

- 1 teaspoon of cinnamon
- 6 packets of Splenda No Calorie Sweetener

Directions:

1. Use a hand mixer to mix all the ingredients in a medium-sized mixing bowl until it becomes smooth
2. Refrigerate for 1 hour before serving

Nutrients Per Serving: Calories 79, Protein 4g, Carbohydrates 9g, Fat 3g, Cholesterol 8mg, Sodium 78mg, Potassium 80mg, Phosphorus 57mg, Fiber 0.1g

Tips:

- Serve either with a low cut-up potassium fruit or low-sodium crackers
- The flavor of yogurt this dip uses need not be vanilla. However, using other flavors of yogurt may alter the nutrient contents and the dip's color
- Dairy is contained in this dip. However, small amounts are okay for patients with dialysis only when potassium and phosphorus levels are well controlled. Nonetheless, consult with your dietitian
- The protein content of Greek yogurt per serving is higher than other yogurts

Homemade Flour Tortilla Chips

Suitable For: CKD non-dialysis, dialysis, and diabetes

Preparation Time: 10 minutes; **Cooking Time:** 10 minutes; **Servings:** 6; **Serving Size:** 8 chips

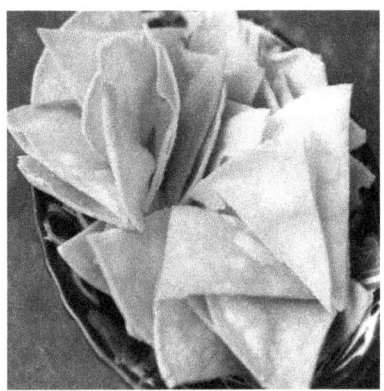

Ingredients:

- 6 flour of 6-inch tortillas
- ½ cup of canola oil

Directions:

- Cut each tortilla into eight pieces, wedge-shaped.
- Use a heavy skillet to heat the oil, using enough to cover ¼ inch of the skillet
- Add the pieces of the tortilla when the oil is hot, then toss until it becomes golden brown and crisp
- Remove chips, draining oil on paper towels
- Store chips in a container until ready to serve

Nutrients Per Serving: Calories 163, Protein 2g, Carbohydrates 14g, Fat 11g, Cholesterol 0g, Sodium 200mg, Potassium 41mg, Phosphorus 54mg, Fiber 0.7g

Cucumber Cheese Sandwich Spread

Suitable For: CKD non-dialysis, dialysis, and diabetes

Preparation Time: 15 minutes; **Cooking Time:** 0 minutes; **Servings:** 16; **Serving Size:** 2 tablespoons

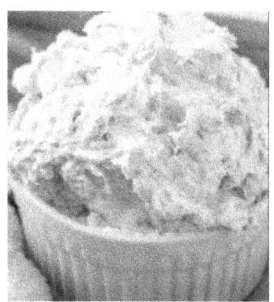

Ingredients:

- 8 ounces of cream cheese
- 1 medium-sized cucumber
- 1 teaspoon of onion
- ¼ teaspoon of salt (or exclude to reduce sodium)
- 1 teaspoon of mayonnaise
- ⅛ teaspoon of green food coloring

Directions:

1. Set out the cream cheese to soften

2. Peel, seed, and mince the cucumber, then set aside. Mince the onion
3. Use a small bowl to mix the cream cheese, onion, salt, mayonnaise, and green food coloring. Blend until it becomes smooth
4. Fold the cucumber into the mixture until it blends evenly

Nutrients Per Serving: Calories 54, Protein 1g, Carbohydrates 1g, Fat 5g, Cholesterol 16mg, Sodium 80mg, Potassium 48mg, Phosphorus 20mg, Fiber 0.1g

Tips:

- The cream cheese analysis is for regular cream cheese. Fat-free cream cheese also works great
- The cucumber cream cheese spread is great for sandwiches on white bread. Cut off the crust from the bread, then cut the sandwiches into triangles for a delightful appetizer. It is also good to use on low-salt saltine crackers

Cold Veggie Pizza

Suitable For: CKD non-dialysis, dialysis, and diabetes

Preparation Time: 10 minutes; **Cooking Time:** 15 minutes; **Servings:** 20; **Serving Size:** 1 piece, 2¼ x 2½ -inch

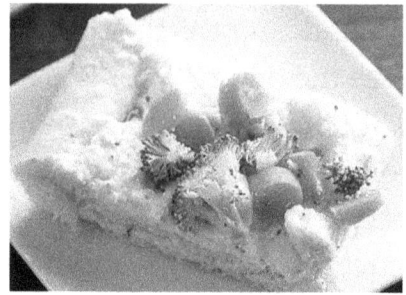

Ingredients:

- 16 ounces of crescent roll dough
- ½ cup of sour cream
- 1 cup of whipped cream cheese
- 2 tablespoons of low-fat Ranch salad dressing
- ¼ teaspoon of garlic powder
- 1 cup of broccoli florets
- 1 medium-sized carrot
- ½ medium-sized cucumber
- ½ cup of red onion
- ½ cup of cherry tomatoes

Directions:

1. Preheat the oven to 350º F.
2. Use a non- stick cooking spray to spray a 13 x 9 x 2-inch baking pan
3. Roll out the packs of the crescent rolls onto the baking pan, then form into a flat single dough surface. Bake for about 10 to 15 minutes, and allow it to cool for about 10 to 15 minutes

4. Beat the cream cheese and sour cream in a bowl until it becomes smooth. Add and stir in the ranch salad dressing and garlic powder, then evenly spread the mixture over the baked crescent
5. Chop the broccoli, cucumber, carrot, and onion, and slice then cherry tomatoes into half
6. Place the chopped vegetables on top of the cream cheese mixture
7. Cover the pizza using a plastic wrap and refrigerate until time to serve.
8. Cut 4 even vertical slices and 5 horizontal slices for 20 pieces

Nutrients Per Serving: Calories 128, Protein 3g, Carbohydrates 11g, Fat 9g, Cholesterol 12mg, Sodium 228mg, Potassium 90mg, Phosphorus 53mg, Fiber 0.4g

Apple Filled Crepes

Suitable For: CKD non-dialysis, dialysis, and diabetes

Preparation Time: 10 minutes; **Cooking Time:** 40 minutes; Servings: 6; Serving Size: 1 crepe

Ingredients:

- 4 egg yolks
- 2 whole eggs
- ½ cup of sugar
- 1 cup of all-purpose

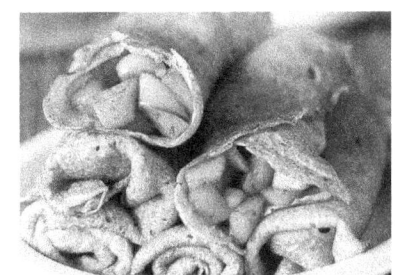

flour
- ¼ cup of oil
- 2 cups of milk
- 4 apples
- ½ cup of brown sugar
- ½ teaspoon of cinnamon
- ½ teaspoon of nutmeg
- ½ cup of unsalted butter

Directions:

Preparing crepe batter:

1. Using a bowl, add and mix the egg yolks, whole eggs, flour, sugar, oil, and milk until the batter becomes smooth and free of lumps
2. Use a small non-stick skillet and heat skillet over medium heat. Spray with cooking spray
3. Use either a ¼ cup or a 2-ounce ladle to spoon 1 scoop of each batter into the heated pan. Swirl pan to spread the crepe batter across the pan
4. Cook for about 20 seconds, flip the crepe, then cook for an additional 10 seconds. Set the crepes aside.
5. Repeat with remaining batter

Preparing filling and assembling crepe:

1. Peel and slice the apples into 12 pieces each.

2. Heat a medium-sized saute pan, melt in the butter, then add the brown sugar
3. Add in the apples, cinnamon, and nutmeg, then cook the apples until it becomes tender but not mushy. Put aside to cool
4. Fill the center of each crepe with about two tablespoons of the apple filling and roll into a log or fold each crepe in quarters with a portion of the apple filling on the side

Nutrients Per Serving: Calories 315, Protein 5g, Carbohydrates 40g, Sodium 356mg, Potassium 160mg, Phosphorus 103mg, Fiber 15g

Tips:

- The crepes can be prepared a day before or even hours in advance. Just cover the crepe with a plastic wrap, refrigerate, and microwave when you are ready to serve.

Apple Rice Salad

Suitable For: CKD non-dialysis, dialysis, and diabetes

Preparation Time: 10 minutes; **Cooking Time:** 10 minutes; **Servings:** 4; **Serving Size:** 1 cup

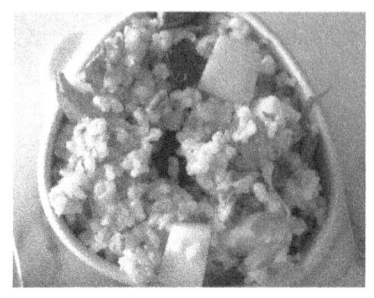

Ingredients:

- 2 cups of cooked, chilled rice
- 2 cups of 2 medium-sized chopped apples
- 2 cup of thinly sliced celery
- 2 tablespoons of unsalted shelled sunflower seeds
- 2 tablespoons of balsamic vinegar
- 1 tablespoon of olive oil
- 2 teaspoons of honey
- 2 teaspoons of brown or dijon mustard
- 2 teaspoons of shredded orange peel
- 1 clove of minced garlic

Directions:

1. Using a large bowl, thoroughly mix the rice, apple, celery, and sunflower seeds
2. Using a small bowl, stir the remaining ingredients together, then pour into the rice mixture, tossing lightly to coat
3. Serve right away, or cover and place in the refrigerator for up to 24 hours

Nutrients Per Serving: Calories 212, Protein 4g, Carbohydrates 42g, Fat 4g, Sodium 74mg, Potassium 206mg, Phosphorus 79mg

Fiesta Pinwheels

Suitable For: CKD non-dialysis, dialysis, and diabetes

Preparation Time: 1hr; **Cooking Time**: 0 minutes; **Servings:** 12; **Serving Size:** 4 pieces, 1-inch each

Ingredients:

- 4 ounces of canned chopped green chilies
- ½ teaspoon of garlic powder

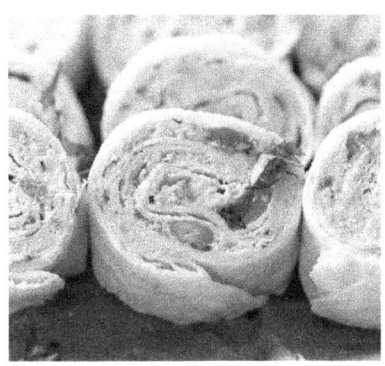

- ½ teaspoon of cumin
- ½ teaspoon of chili powder
- 4 tablespoons of green onion
- 8 ounces of cream cheese
- 6 flour of 8-inch tortillas

Directions:

1. Set out the cream cheese to soften, and slice the green onion
2. Use a bowl and mix the green chilies, spices and green onions
3. Stir in the softened cream cheese
4. Spread the cream cheese mixture on each tortilla with ¼ inch edge left uncovered

5. Roll-up the tortillas on a plastic wrap or use a toothpick to hold it down, Refrigerate for about one hour
6. Remove plastic wrap and cut the rolls into 1-inch pieces and serve

Nutrients Per Serving: Calories 148, Protein 3g, Carbohydrates 16g, Fat 8g, Cholesterol 21mg, Sodium 260mg, Potassium 73mg, Phosphorus 52mg, Fiber 0.9g

Brie with Cranberry Chutney

Suitable For: CKD non-dialysis, dialysis, and diabetes

Preparation Time: 10 minutes; **Cooking Time:** 45 minutes; **Servings:** 10; **Serving Size:** ¾-ounce Brie, 2 teaspoons chutney and 3 low-sodium crackers

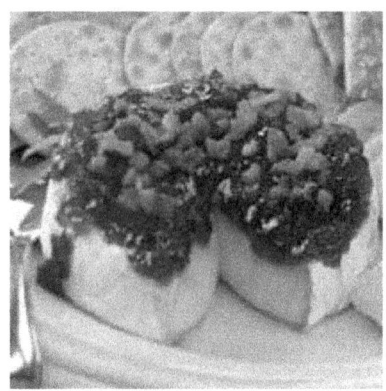

Ingredients:

- 12 ounces of fresh cranberries

- ⅓ cup of water
- ½ cup of sugar
- ½ cup of brown sugar
- 1 teaspoon of dry mustard
- 1 teaspoon cloves
- 1 teaspoon of cinnamon
- 1 teaspoon of nutmeg
- 1 teaspoon of allspice
- 8 ounces of Brie cheese
- 30 low sodium crackers

Directions:

1. Preheat oven to 350° F
2. Wash and drain the fresh cranberries. Using a large skillet and over medium heat, heat the water for about 5 minutes, then add the cranberries. Heat for an additional 5 minutes just until the cranberries begin to burst
3. Add in the white and brown sugar, add the spices and stir slightly
4. Remove chutney from the heat, and allow it to cool
5. Take off the wheel of Brie from its wrapper, leave ½ inch border of rind over the wheel, then cut out a circle. Lift the rind off from the center to reveal the Brie inside

6. Use a baking sheet and place the Brie on it. Place Brie and heat in the oven just until the Brie cheese becomes soft with the top slightly melted
7. Remove the Brie from the oven and place on a platter
8. Spread the chutney over the Brie and serve with of low-sodium crackers

Nutrients Per Serving: Calories 204, Protein 6g, Carbohydrate 27g, Fat 8g, Cholesterol 28mg, Sodium 184mg, Potassium 118mg, Phosphorus 65mg, Fiber 1.9g

Tips:

- Low-sodium crackers are recommended to keep the sodium levels low
- Cranberry Chutney can be stored in the refrigerator for up to three days before serving
- Cranberry Chutney can also be used with turkey, pork or lamb

Lumpia Filipino Spring Rolls

Suitable For: CKD non-dialysis, dialysis, and diabetes

Preparation Time: 25 minutes; **Cooking Time:** 25 minutes; **Servings:** 15; **Serving Size:** 2 pieces lumpia

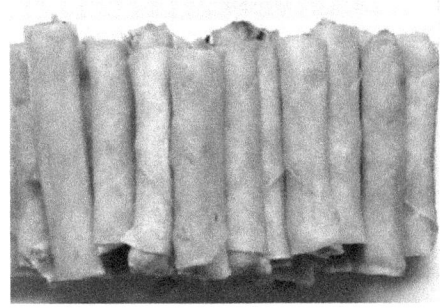

Ingredients:

- 2 cloves of garlic
- ½ cup of white onion
- 2 green onions
- 1pound of ground pork
- 1 tablespoon of canola oil
- 1 cup of coleslaw mix
- 1 teaspoon of ground black pepper
- 1 teaspoon of garlic powder
- 1 teaspoon of reduced-sodium soy sauce
- 30 lumpia wrappers
- 2 cups of peanut oil for frying

Directions:

1. Mince garlic, and slice the white and green onion
2. Brown the ground pork in a large skillet. Remove the pork and put aside, allowing it to drain on paper towels

3. Use canola oil to coat the skillet, then add the garlic, white onion and sauté until the onions are translucent
4. Pour in the coleslaw mix, the green onions, and the browned pork. Stir to mix and continue cooking
5. Sprinkle pepper, garlic powder, and the sauce over the mixture and stir. Remove from the heat and set aside to cool
6. Place diagonally, two tablespoons of the mixture from step 5 near a corner of the lumpia wrapper, and leave space at both ends. Fold the side closer to you over the mixture, then fold both sides and roll, keep it tight. Seal by using water to moisten an edge of the wrapper to seal.
7. Repeat using the remaining wrappers. Also, ensure the rolls are covered with a plastic wrap to prevent drying
8. Over medium heat, heat a deep skillet, then add peanut oil to a depth of ½ inch, and heat for about 5 minutes. Slide-in 3 to 4 lumpia into the heated oil, and fry for 1 to 2 minutes, until it becomes golden brown
9. Drain oil on paper towels, then serve

Nutrients Per Serving: Calories 257, Protein 11g, Carbohydrates 31g, Fat 10g, Cholesterol 44mg, Sodium 203mg, Potassium 158mg, Phosphorus 90mg, Fiber 1.1g

Tips:

- Lumpia wrappers can be obtained in most Asian markets. However, if unavailable, use won ton wrappers
- Put the seam down first when frying the lumpia - it helps seal them better
- Ground pork can be substituted for ground turkey or chicken

Maple Trail Mix

Suitable For: CKD non-dialysis, dialysis, and diabetes

Preparation Time: 10 minutes; **Cooking Time:** 30 minutes; **Servings:** 24; **Serving Size:** 1 cup

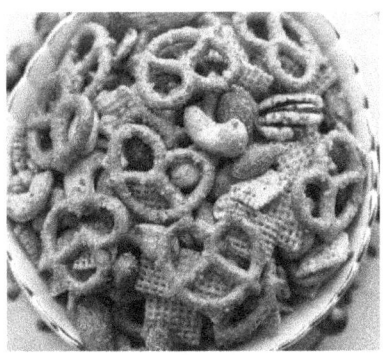

Ingredients:

- 3 cups of Golden Grahams cereal
- 5 cups of Rice Chex cereal

- 10 ounces of Cinnamon Teddy Grahams snack cookies
- 6 ounces of Pretzel Crisps
- ½ of cup unsalted butter
- ⅓ cup of dark brown sugar
- ¼ cup of honey
- ¼ cup of maple syrup
- 5 ounces of dried sweetened cranberries
- 3 ounces of Crispy Granny Smith Apple Chips

Directions:

1. Using a large bowl, combine and mix the Golden Grahams, Rice Chex, Teddy Grahams and pretzels
2. Use a small saucepan to melt the butter, add the brown sugar, honey, and maple syrup, then cook on low heat until the sugar melt
3. Stir in the cereal mixture from step 1 until all the pieces have been coated
4. Preheat the oven to 325° F
5. Make three jelly roll pans by lining with foil. Spray foil with cooking spray (can be done in a batch of 3) and spread evenly over the pans with the cereal mixture. Bake for about 20 minutes.
6. Add and mix the cranberries and Apple Chips, and divide among the pans and stir
7. Bake for an additional 5 minutes, then allow to cool before storing in an airtight container

Nutrients Per Serving: Calories 262, Protein 3g, Carbohydrates 47g, Fat 9g, Cholesterol 11mg, Sodium 178mg, Potassium 84mg, Phosphorus 66mg, Fiber 1.8g

Tips:

- If Pretzel Crisps are not available, you can substitute for a 10-ounce mini pretzel twists
- If you have diabetes, reduce the serving size to 1/2 cup for a reduced carbohydrate snack

Party Deviled Eggs

Suitable For: CKD non-dialysis, dialysis, and diabetes

Preparation Time: 10 minutes; **Cooking Time:** 15 minutes; **Servings:** 2; **Serving Size:** 2 halves

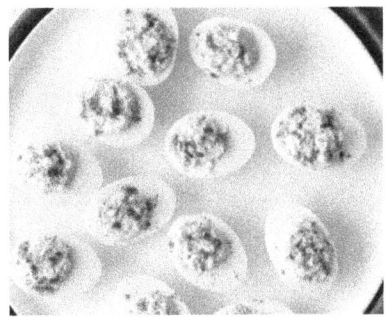

Ingredients:

- 2 large eggs
- 2 teaspoons of canned pimento

- ½ teaspoon of dry mustard
- 2 tablespoons of mayonnaise
- ½ teaspoon of black pepper
- ⅛ teaspoon of paprika

Directions:

1. Hard boil the eggs, drain water and set aside to cool
2. Crack the egg shells, and peel carefully under cool running water, then cut the eggs in half lengthwise. Transfer the yolk to a small bowl, and place the egg whites on a serving platter.
3. Mash the yolk with a fork, dice the pimento, then mix all together with the mustard, mayonnaise, and pepper
4. Place the mixture inside the egg whites in two equal parts
5. Spread the eggs with the paprika and serve

Nutrients Per Serving: Calories 137, Protein 6g, Carbohydrates 1g, Fat 11g, Cholesterol 353mg, Sodium 176mg, Potassium 66mg, Phosphorus 94mg, Fiber 0.3g

Chapter 6

Vegetables

Carrot Casserole

Suitable For: CKD non-dialysis, dialysis, and diabetes

Preparation Time: 10 minutes; **Cooking Time:** 25 minutes; **Servings:** 8; **Serving Size:** ½ cup

Ingredients:

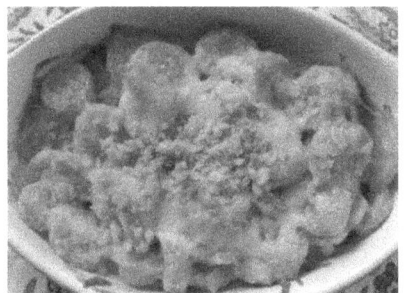

- 1 pound of carrots
- 12 low-sodium Ritz crackers or any low sodium substitutes
- 2 tablespoons of butter
- 2 tablespoons of onion
- ¼ teaspoon of salt (or exclude to reduce sodium)
- ¼ teaspoon of black pepper
- ⅓ cup of shredded cheddar cheese

Directions:

1. Preheat oven to 350º F
2. Peel the carrots and cut into ¼ inch rounds. Use a large saucepan and place the carrots in it. Heat over medium to high heat and cook until it

becomes soft enough to mash. Drain, reserving ⅓-cup liquid
3. Mash the carrots until they become smooth. Set aside in a bowl
4. Crush the crackers, melt the butter, and mince the onion. Stir in the crackers, onion, butter, salt, pepper, and the reserved liquid into the mashed carrots
5. Transfer to a small greased casserole dish, and sprinkle the shredded cheese on top. Bake for about 15 minutes and serve hot

Nutrients Per Serving: Calories 94, Protein 2g, Carbohydrates 9g, Fat 6g, Cholesterol 13mg, Sodium 174mg, Potassium 153mg, Phosphorus 47mg, Fiber 1.8g

Zucchini French Fries

Suitable For: CKD non-dialysis, dialysis, and diabetes

Preparation Time: 15 minutes; **Cooking Time:** 20 minutes; **Servings:** 6; **Serving Size:** 7-8 pieces

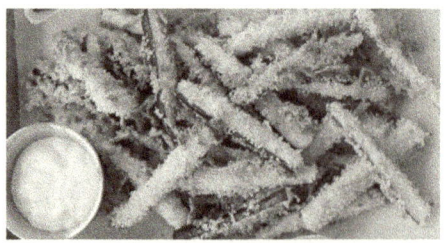

Ingredients:

- 2 medium-sized zucchini
- 1 cup of low-fat milk
- 2 large eggs
- ¾ cup of cornstarch
- ¾ cup of dry unseasoned bread crumbs
- 3 teaspoons of dry Original Hidden Valley Ranch Salad Dressing and Seasoning Mix
- 1 teaspoon of Tabasco hot sauce (optional)
- ½ cup of canola oil

Directions:

1. Peel and cut the zucchini into ¾ inch sticks, 4-inch long. Rinse, then pat dry
2. Mix the milk and eggs in a medium bowl until it is well blended, then stir in the Tabasco hot sauce. Set aside
3. Use a bowl, then combine and mix the cornstarch, bread crumbs, and the dry Ranch salad dressing. Set aside
4. Heat oil over a high heat frying pan
5. Dip the sticks of zucchini into the egg mixture, then roll each of the pieces into the bread crumb mixture
6. Place the mixed zucchini mixture into the oil, flipping regularly. Fry for about 3 minutes or until it turns golden brown
7. Drain on paper towels, and serve warm

Nutrients Per Serving: Calories 252, Protein 5g, Carbohydrates 22g, Fat 16g, Cholesterol 64mg, Sodium 216mg, Potassium 263mg, Phosphorus 105mg, Fiber 1.0g

Marinated Fresh Vegetables

Suitable For: CKD non-dialysis, dialysis, and diabetes

Preparation Time: 10 minutes; **Cooking Time:** 15 minutes; **Servings:** 12; **Serving Size:** ¾ cup

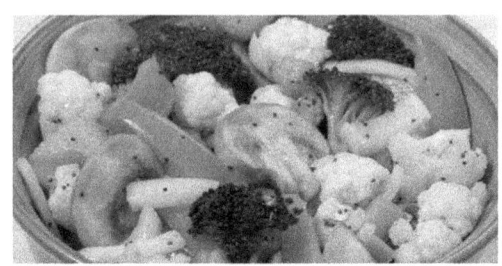

Ingredients:

- 3 cups of broccoli florets
- 3 cups of cauliflower florets
- 2 cups of sliced mushrooms
- 1 cup of green bell pepper
- 1 cup of celery
- ½ cup of onion
- ½ cup of sugar
- 2 teaspoons of dry mustard
- ½ teaspoon of salt (or exclude to reduce sodium)
- ½ cup of vinegar

- 1 cup of olive oil
- 1 tablespoon of poppy seeds

Directions:

1. Cut the broccoli and cauliflower into pieces (bite-sized), cut the peppers and celery, then chop the onion
2. Combine and mix in a bowl the broccoli, cauliflower, mushrooms, pepper, and celery
3. In another bowl, combine and mix the remaining ingredients to prepare the marinade, then pour over the vegetables. Refrigerate at about 3 hours before serving
4. Using a slotted spoon, remove the vegetables from the marinade before serving

Nutrients Per Serving: Calories 174, Protein 2g, Carbohydrates 10g, Fat 14g, Cholesterol 0mg, Sodium 112mg, Potassium 250mg, Phosphorus 50mg, Fiber 1.9g

Tips:

- Adjusting the serving size to ½ cup would reduce the potassium serving to 167 mg
- Leftovers can be stored in the refrigerator for 5 days

Ratatouille

Suitable For: CKD non-dialysis, and diabetes

Preparation Time: 10 minutes; **Cooking Time:** 50 minutes; **Servings:** 16; **Serving Size:** ½ cup

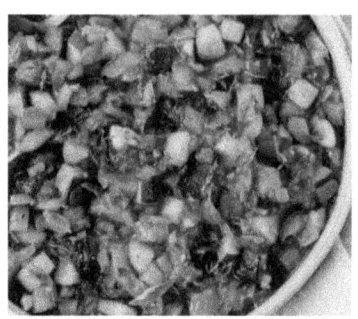

Ingredients:

- 2 cups of onion
- 2 cups of zucchini squash
- 3 cups of yellow crookneck squash
- 1 medium-sized eggplant
- 2 medium of carrots
- 1 green bell pepper
- 1 yellow bell pepper
- 1 red bell pepper
- 4 garlic cloves
- 2 tablespoons of olive oil
- 1 cup of canned tomatoes
- 1 tablespoon of fresh basil
- 1 tablespoon of fresh oregano
- 1 tablespoon of fresh rosemary

- 1 tablespoon of fresh thyme
- 1 tablespoon of fresh sage
- 1 tablespoon of black pepper
- 8 tablespoons of grated parmesan cheese

Directions:

1. Dice the onion, squash, carrots, eggplant, and bell peppers. Also, mince the garlic cloves
2. Add olive oil to a large skillet, and add in the garlic cloves, herbs, black pepper, and the carrots
3. Cook for about 2 minutes, then add in the rest of the vegetables, excluding the tomatoes
4. Sauté properly, and frequently stirring for about 10–15 minutes or until the vegetables become semi-tender
5. Add in the tomatoes and parmesan cheese. Mix thoroughly
5. Cover and simmer for approximately ½ hour

Nutrients Per Serving: Calories 54, Protein 3g, Carbohydrates 6g, Fat 3g, Cholesterol 2mg, Sodium 84mg, Potassium 302mg, Phosphorus 58mg, Fiber 2.4g

Tips:

- If you are using the dried herbs rather than fresh, reduce to 1 teaspoon instead of 1 tablespoon
- Ratatouille can be used as a side dish
- Extra portions can be refrigerated for a later dish

Roasted Rosemary Cauliflower

Suitable For: CKD non-dialysis, dialysis, and diabetes

Preparation Time: 5 minutes; **Cooking Time:** 25 minutes; **Servings:** 9; **Serving Size:** ⅔ cup

Ingredients:

- 6 cups of cauliflower florets
- 1 tablespoon of fresh rosemary
- 1½ tablespoons of olive oil
- ¼ teaspoon of salt (or remove to reduce sodium)
- ¼ teaspoon black pepper

Directions:

1. Preheat oven to 450° F
2. Cut the cauliflower florets into pieces (bite-sized), and chop the rosemary
3. Toss the cauliflower with the remaining ingredients in a large bowl
4. Spread the seasoned cauliflower on a baking sheet (ungreased)
5. Roast for about 15 minutes, then remove from the oven and stir
6. Continue roasting for an additional 10 minutes or until the cauliflower becomes tender and slightly browned

Nutrients Per Serving: Calories 32, Protein 1g, Carbohydrates 2g, Fat 2g, Cholesterol 0mg, Sodium 80mg, Potassium 204mg, Phosphorus 30mg

Tips:

- Apply caution when taking out the baking sheet from the oven to stir the cauliflower

Seasoned Cabbage Steaks

Suitable For: CKD non-dialysis, dialysis, and diabetes

Preparation Time: 10 minutes; **Cooking Time:** 15 minutes; **Servings:** 6; **Serving Size:** 1 cabbage steak

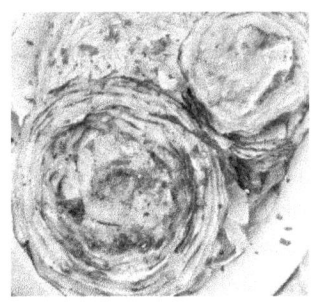

Ingredients:

- 1 medium-sized cabbage head
- 2 tablespoons of olive oil
- ½ teaspoon of black pepper
- 1 tablespoon of salt-free herb seasoning
- 1 tablespoon of fresh dill weed

Directions:

1. Preheat oven to 350° F
2. Slice the cabbage head into six 1-inch thick pieces
3. Arrange the sliced cabbage pieces on a baking sheet, drizzling with olive oil. Sprinkle the herb seasoning and dill weed over the cabbage. Cover with foil
4. Bake for about 45 minutes, then remove the foil and allow the cabbage steaks to brown in the oven for an extra 15 minutes

Nutrients Per Serving: Calories 90, Protein 2g, Carbohydrates 9g, Fat 5g, Cholesterol 0mg, Sodium 26mg, Potassium 267mg, Phosphorus 38mg

Tips:

- Use ½ cup of Greek yogurt and an extra chopped fresh dill weed to prepare a sauce to serve with the cabbage steaks (if desired)

Stuffed Zucchini Boats

Suitable For: CKD non-dialysis, dialysis, and diabetes

Preparation Time: 10 minutes; **Cooking Time:** 25 minutes; **Servings:** 4; **Serving Size:** ½ zucchini with stuffing

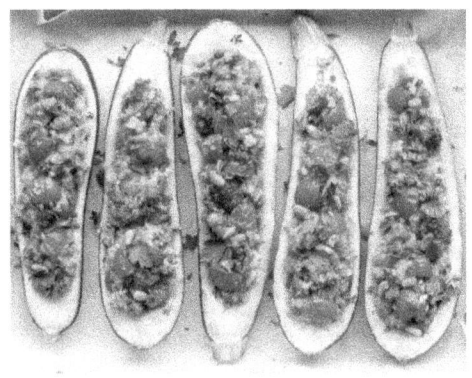

Ingredients:

- 2 medium-sized zucchini
- 4 slices of white bread
- ¼ teaspoon of ground sage
- 1 teaspoon of onion powder
- 1 teaspoon of original Mrs. Dash seasoning blend
- 1 teaspoon of salt-free lemon pepper
- 1 teaspoon of dill weed

Directions:

1. Pre-heat oven to 375° F
2. Cut the zucchini into half lengthwise. Use a spoon to scoop out the seeds to form a trench in each half of the zucchini
3. Place the zucchini in a pot of boiling water, boiling for about 3 to 5 minutes
4. Toast two slices of bread while the zucchini cooks
5. Place the toasted and the two untoasted slices of bread in a food processor to make bread crumbs

6. Add all the seasonings to the bread crumbs and mix properly
7. Add ½ cup of the cooking water (zucchini) and blend using a fork for consistency in stuffing
8. Remove the zucchini from the water, placing it in an 8 x 8-inch baking dish. Peel side down
9. Use a spoon to stuff into each half of zucchini, and bake for 20 minutes before serving

Nutrients Per Serving: Calories 82, Protein 3g, Carbohydrates 15g, Fat 1g, Cholesterol 0mg, Sodium 180mg, Potassium 276mg, Phosphorus 63mg, Fiber 1.7g

Spanish Vegetable Paella

Suitable For: CKD non-dialysis, dialysis, and diabetes

Preparation Time: 10 minutes; **Cooking Time:** 20 minutes; **Servings**: 8; **Serving Size:** 1¼ cup

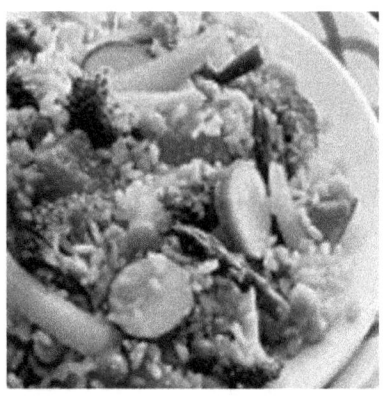

Ingredients:

- 2 cups of asparagus
- 3 cups of broccoli florets
- 1 tablespoon of olive oil
- 1 cup of green bell pepper
- 1¼ of cup zucchini
- ½ cup of onion
- 2 cups of uncooked brown rice
- ½ teaspoon of salt (or exclude to reduce sodium)
- ½ teaspoon saffron

Directions:

1. Chop the bell pepper, zucchini, and onion
2. Cook the rice in boiling water until it becomes tender, then drain
3. Fill a saucepan of 2-quart with enough water to cover the asparagus and broccoli. Cook the asparagus and broccoli for 4 minutes or until it becomes crisp-tender, then drain
4. Heat oil over medium heat using a 10-inch skillet. Cook asparagus, broccoli, rice, bell pepper, zucchini and onion in oil for 5 minutes. Stir periodically until the onion becomes crisp-tender
5. Stir in the remaining ingredients and cook for an additional 5 minutes. Frequently stir until cooked

Nutrients Per Serving: Calories 146, Protein 5g, Carbohydrates 26g, Fat 2g, Cholesterol 0mg, Sodium 150mg, Potassium 305mg, Phosphorus 89mg, Fiber 1.8g

Tips:

- Serving size can be reduced to ¾ cup if you're on a low potassium diet
- ¼ teaspoon of ground turmeric can be substituted for saffron

Yellow Hearty Squash Casserole

Suitable For: CKD non-dialysis, dialysis, and diabetes

Preparation Time: 10 minutes; **Cooking Time:** 50 minutes; **Servings:** B **Serving Size:** ⅛ of casserole

Ingredients:

- 6 slices of whole wheat bread
- 4 medium-sized yellow squash
- ½ cup of water
- ½ cup of carrots
- ½ cup of sweet onion
- ¼ teaspoon salt (or exclude to reduce sodium)
- 2 tablespoon of flaxseed

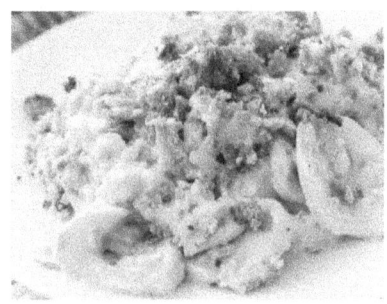

- 2 eggs
- 2 tablespoons of unsalted butter

Directions:

1. Preheat oven to 350°F
2. Process the bread in a food processor until it crumbles
3. Slice the squash, then microwave with water for about 16 minutes or until it becomes tender. Drain the squash using a colander
4. Grate the carrots, chop the onion, then combine the squash, carrots, onion, salt, one tablespoon of flaxseed, and eggs. Mix thoroughly
5. Stir in ½ of the bread crumbs
6. Use a non-stick cooking spray to spray a 9-inch square pan. Pour the mixture into the baking pan, and set aside
7. Melt the butter, and add along with the remaining bread crumbs and flaxseed to prepare the topping. Mix properly
8. Spread the topping over the casserole mixture, then bake for about 30 minutes or until the topping begins to brown

Nutrients Per Serving: Calories 130, Protein 6g, Carbohydrates 15g, Fat 5g, Cholesterol 54mg, Sodium 195mg, Potassium 328mg, Phosphorus 111mg, Fiber 2.8g

Bowtie Pasta with Veggie Crumbles and Kale

Suitable For: CKD non-dialysis, dialysis, and diabetes

Preparation Time: 10 minutes; **Cooking Time:** 35 minutes; **Servings:** 6; **Serving Size:** 1⅓ cups

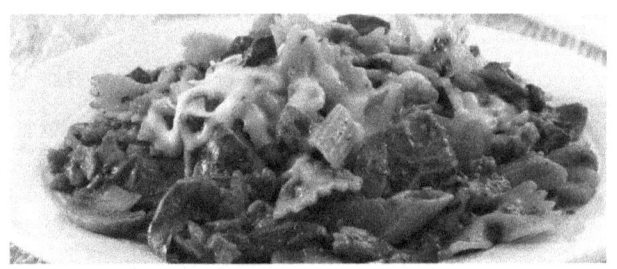

Ingredients:

- 1 cup of onion
- 1 tablespoon of olive oil
- 12 ounces of frozen veggie crumbles
- ⅓ cup of water
- 2 teaspoons of Italian seasoning blend
- 4 cups of low-sodium vegetable broth
- 8 ounces of bowtie pasta
- 2 cups of kale
- ⅛ teaspoon of red chili flakes
- ½ cup of plain, low-fat Greek yogurt

Directions:

1. Slice the onion and kale

2. Heat the olive oil in a large skillet over medium heat, then sauté the onion until it becomes tender. Stir in the veggie crumbles, water, and the Italian seasoning. Cover and cook for about 4 minutes or until it crumbles
3. Pour into the mixture, a 2-½ cups of vegetable broth and bring to a boil
4. Add the pasta, cook, and stir over medium-high heat for about 10 to 12 minutes or until the broth becomes absorbed. Add the remaining broth, chili flakes, and kale. Cook over medium heat for about 14 minutes or until the pasta is done
5. Remove the skillet from heat, stirring in the Greek yogurt. Serve hot

Nutrients Per Serving: Calories 280, Protein 18g, Carbohydrates 39g, Fat 6g, Cholesterol 2mg, Sodium 350mg, Potassium 340mg, Phosphorus 203mg, Fiber 6.1g

Tips:

- Soy protein products differ to a large extent per the potassium content. Always check the product label for potassium content
- Several soy-based vegetarian protein products contain a large amount of sodium. Use other low-sodium substitute ingredients in your recipes to keep the total sodium low.

Chapter 7

Seafood

Citrus Grilled Glazed Salmon

Suitable For: CKD non-dialysis, dialysis, and diabetes

Preparation Time: 10 minutes; **Cooking Time:** 20 minutes; **Servings:** 6; **Serving Size:** 3 ounces

Ingredients:

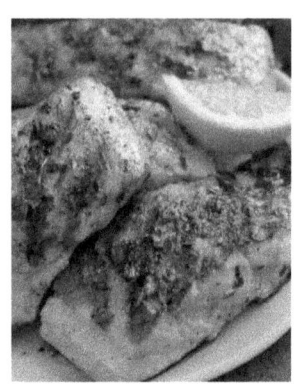

- 2 garlic cloves
- 1½ tablespoons of lemon juice
- 2 tablespoons of olive oil
- 1 tablespoon of unsalted butter
- 1 tablespoon of Dijon mustard
- 2 dashes of cayenne pepper
- 1 teaspoon of dried basil leaves
- 1 teaspoon of dried dill
- 1 tablespoon of capers
- 24 ounces of salmon filet

Directions:

1. Crush the garlic

2. Combine all ingredients in a small saucepan, excluding the salmon, heat to a boil, then reduce the heat to low. Cook for about 5 minutes
3. Preheat grill, then place the salmon with its skin side down on a sheet of foil that is a little bigger than the fish. Fold up the edges so that the sauce remains with the salmon on the grill. Place on top of the grill, the foil and fish, then top the salmon with the sauce mixture from step 2
4. Cover grill and cook for about 12 minutes or until the salmon has cooked (Don't flip the salmon).
5. Cut the salmon into six servings

Nutrients Per Serving: Calories 294, Protein 23g, Carbohydrates 1g, Fat 22g, Cholesterol 68mg, Sodium 190mg, Potassium 439mg, Phosphorus 280 mg, Fiber 0.2g

Tips:

- The recipe analysis is based on farmed Atlantic salmon. Wild Alaskan salmon has little fat content but a little higher both in potassium and phosphorus. However, both are healthy and recommended for a kidney diet
- This recipe can also be cooked in the oven at 350°F for about 10 to 15 minutes or until it is cooked.
- Adjust the serving size if you are on a lower protein diet

Maryland Crab Cakes

Suitable For: CKD non-dialysis, dialysis, and diabetes

Preparation Time: 5 minutes; **Cooking Time:** 15 minutes; **Servings:** 6; **Serving Size:** 1 crab cake

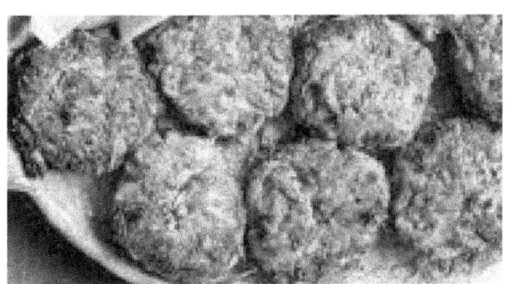

Ingredients:

- 1 pound of lump crab meat
- 1 slice of white bread
- 1 tablespoon of mayonnaise
- 1 teaspoon of yellow mustard
- 1 teaspoon of 30% less sodium Old Bay seasoning
- 1 tablespoon of fresh parsley
- ⅛ teaspoon of cayenne pepper
- 1 large egg
- 2 tablespoons of olive oil

Directions:

1. Pick through the crab meat in a medium bowl, removing any shell pieces
2. Cut the slice of bread into cubes

3. Add in all the ingredients to the except the olive oil. Mix slightly until all the ingredients are combined. Don't over mix
4. Portion out six crab cakes using ⅓ cup, with each portion being ¾ inch thick. Store in the refrigerator for one hour
5. Heat oil or cooking spray in a heavy skillet, and fry both sides of the crab for 5 minutes each or until it becomes browned

Nutrients Per Serving: Calories 158, Protein 17g, Carbohydrates 2g, Fat 9g, Cholesterol 112mg, Sodium 337mg, Potassium 268mg, Phosphorus 177mg, Fiber 0.3g

Tips:

- You can use paprika rather than Old Bay seasoning. With that, sodium is cut further to 274 mg per serving
- The bread can be replaced with ½ cup of crushed saltines, unsalted tops
- Mandarin orange slices garnished with chopped lettuce can be served with it

Tilapia Ceviche

Suitable For: CKD non-dialysis, dialysis, and diabetes

Preparation Time: 2hr 15 minutes; **Cooking Time:** 0 minutes; **Servings:** 8; **Serving Size:** 1 cup with 6 crackers

Ingredients:

- 1½ pounds of fresh tilapia fillets
- 1 cup of red onion
- ½ cup of red bell pepper
- ¼ cup of cilantro
- 1 cup of pineapple
- 2 tablespoons of canola oil
- ¼ teaspoon of black pepper
- 1¼ cups of fresh lime juice
- 48 saltine crackers with unsalted tops

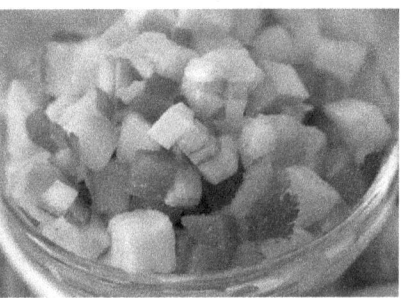

Directions:

1. Chop the onion, bell pepper, and cilantro. Also, dice the pineapple, and cube the tilapia into small chunks
2. Broil tilapia cubes over high heat for about 3 minutes on each side
3. Cool the tilapia for about 5 minutes, then pour the fresh lime juice on top of it, mixing properly.

Ensure all tilapia pieces are coated completely with the lime juice
4. Combine and mix the bell pepper, onion, pineapple, cilantro, black pepper and the canola oil with the broiled tilapia mixture
5. Cover and refrigerate to marinate for about 2 hours
6. Use six saltine crackers with the unsalted tops for each serving

Nutrients Per Serving: Calories 220, Protein 19g, Carbohydrates 20g, Fat 7g, Cholesterol 36mg, Sodium 168mg, Potassium 374mg, Phosphorus 162mg, Fiber 1.3g

Fish Tacos

Suitable For: CKD non-dialysis, dialysis, and diabetes

Preparation Time: 10 minutes; **Cooking Time:** 35 minutes; **Servings:** 6; **Serving Size:** 2 tacos

Ingredients:

- 1½ cup of cabbage

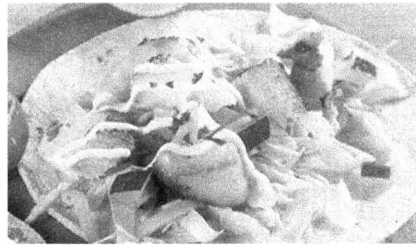

- ½ cup of red onion
- ½ bunch of cilantro
- 1 garlic clove
- 2 limes

- 1 pound of cod fillets
- ½ teaspoon of ground cumin
- ½ teaspoon of chili powder
- ¼ teaspoon of black pepper
- 1 tablespoon of olive oil
- ½ cup of mayonnaise
- ¼ cup of sour cream
- 2 tablespoons of milk
- 12 (6-inch) corn tortillas

Directions:

1. Shred the cabbage, chop the onion and cilantro, and mince the garlic. Set aside
2. Use a dish to place in the fish fillets, then squeeze half a lime juice over the fish. Sprinkle the fish fillets with the minced garlic, cumin, black pepper, chili powder, and olive oil. Turn the fish filets to coat with the marinade, then refrigerate for about 15 to 30 minutes
3. Prepare salsa blanca by mixing the mayonnaise, milk, sour cream, and the other half of the lime juice. Stir to combine, then place in the refrigerator to chill
4. Broil in oven, and cover the broiler pan with aluminum foil. Broil the coated fish fillets for about 10 minutes or until the flesh becomes opaque and white and flakes easily. Remove from the oven, slightly cool, and then flake the fish into bigger pieces

5. Heat the corn tortillas in a pan, one at a time until it becomes soft and warm, then wrap in a dish towel to keep them warm
6. To assemble the tacos, place a piece of the fish on the tortilla, topping with the salsa blanca, cabbage, cilantro, red onion, and the lime wedges.
7. Serve with hot sauce if you desire

Nutrients Per Serving: Calories 363, Protein 18g, Carbohydrates 30g, Fat 19g, Cholesterol 40mg, Sodium 194mg, Potassium 507mg, Phosphorus 327mg, Fiber 4.3g

Tips:

- You can substitute the cod fillet with any firm white fish such as tilapia, catfish, snapper, halibut, and rockfish. They all do well in this recipe
- You can cook the fish on a grill rather than broiling
- Compare brands of hot sauce, and go for the lowest in sodium brand

Jambalaya

Suitable For: CKD non-dialysis, dialysis, and diabetes

Preparation Time: 10 minutes; **Cooking Time:** 1hr 15 minutes; **Servings:** 12; **Serving Size:** 1 cup

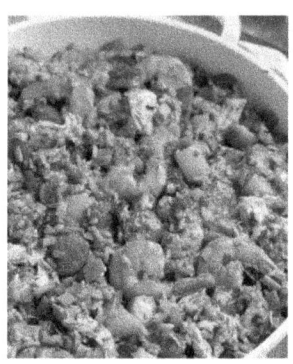

Ingredients:

- 2 cups of onion
- 1 cup of bell pepper
- 2 garlic cloves
- 2 cups of uncooked converted brown rice
- ½ teaspoon of black pepper
- 8 ounces of canned low-sodium tomato sauce
- 2 cups of low-sodium beef broth
- 2 pounds of raw shrimp
- ½ cup of unsalted margarine

Directions:

1. Preheat oven to 350º F

2. Chop the onion, bell pepper, garlic, then peel the shrimp
3. Combine and mix all the ingredients in a large bowl except the margarine
4. Pour into a 9 x 13-inch baking dish and evenly spread out
5. Slice the margarine, placing over the top of the ingredients
6. Cover with foil or lid, and bake for about 1 hr 15 minutes
7. Serve hot

Nutrients Per Serving: Calories 294, Protein 20g, Carbohydrates 31g, Fat 10g, Cholesterol 137mg, Sodium 186mg, Potassium 300mg, Phosphorus 197mg, Fiber 0.8g

Tips:

- Converted rice is also known as parboiled rice. One popular brand of such rice is Uncle Ben's converted brown rice

Asparagus Shrimp Linguini

Suitable For: CKD non-dialysis, and dialysis

Preparation Time: 10 minutes; **Cooking Time:** 35 minutes; **Servings:** 4; **Serving Size:** 1½ cup

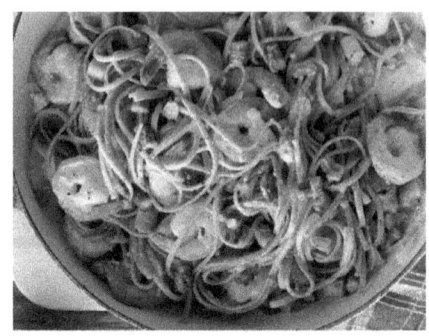

Ingredients:

- 8 ounces of uncooked linguini
- 1 tablespoon of olive oil
- 1¾ cups of asparagus
- ½ cup of unsalted butter
- 2 garlic cloves
- 3 ounces of cream cheese
- 2 tablespoons of fresh parsley
- ¾ teaspoon of dried basil
- ⅔ cup of dry white wine
- ½ pound of peeled and cooked shrimp

Directions:

1. Preheat oven to 350° F
2. Cook the linguini in boiling water until it becomes tender, then drain
3. Place the asparagus on a baking sheet, then spread two tablespoons of oil over the asparagus. Bake for about 7 to 8 minutes or until it is tender

4. Remove baked asparagus from the oven and place it on a plate. Cut the asparagus into pieces of medium-sized once cooled
5. Mince the garlic and chop the parsley
6. Melt ½ cup of butter in a large skillet with the minced garlic
7. Stir in the cream cheese, mixing as it melts
8. Stir in the parsley and basil, then simmer for about 5 minutes. Mix either in boiling water or dry white wine, stirring until the sauce becomes smooth
9. Add the cooked shrimp and asparagus, then stir and heat until it is evenly warm
10. Toss the cooked pasta with the sauce and serve

Nutrients Per Serving: Calories 544, Protein 21g, Carbohydrates 43g, Fat 32g, Cholesterol 188mg, Sodium 170mg, Potassium 402mg, Phosphorus 225mg, Fiber 2.4g

Tips:

- Cooked and peeled frozen shrimp are sold by most grocery stores
- Using dry white wine instead of boiling water provides additional flavor. However, you may choose to use water instead

Tuna Noodle Casserole

Suitable For: CKD non-dialysis, dialysis, and diabetes

Preparation Time: 10 minutes; **Cooking Time:** 35 minutes; **Servings:** 2; **Serving Size:** 2 cups

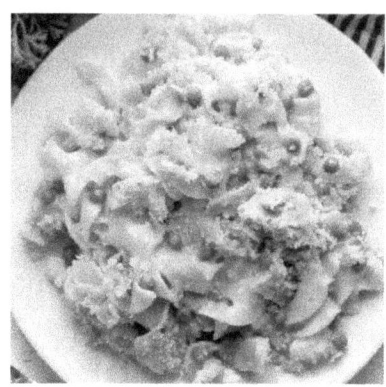

Ingredients:

- 2 ounces of wide uncooked egg noodles
- 5 ounces of canned tuna in water
- ½ cup of sour cream
- ¼ cup of cottage cheese
- ½ cup of fresh sliced mushrooms
- ½ cup of frozen green peas
- 1 tablespoon of unsalted butter
- ¼ cup of unseasoned bread crumbs

Directions:

1. Preheat oven to 350° F

2. Boil egg noodles based on the package instructions and drain. Also, drain and flake the tuna
3. Combine and mix the sour cream, cottage cheese, mushrooms, tuna, and peas in a medium bowl
4. Stir the drained noodle into the tuna mixture, and place in a small casserole dish that has been sprayed with a non-stick cooking spray
5. Melt butter, stir into the bread crumbs, then sprinkle over the mixture of noodles in step 4
6. Bake for about 20 to 25 minutes or until the bread crumbs start to brown
7. Divide into two and serve

Nutrients Per Serving: Calories 415, Protein 22g, Carbohydrates 39g, Fat 19g, Cholesterol 88mg, Sodium 266mg, Potassium 400mg, Phosphorus 306mg, Fiber 3.2g

Tips:

- Leftovers can be stored in the refrigerator for 2 to 3 days

Oven-Fried Southern Style Catfish

Suitable For: CKD non-dialysis, dialysis, and diabetes

Preparation Time: 10 minutes; **Cooking Time:** 35 minutes; **Servings:** 4; **Serving Size:** 3 ounces

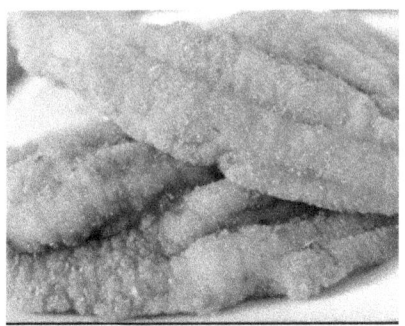

Ingredients:

- 1 egg white
- ½ cup of all-purpose flour
- ¼ cup of cornmeal
- ¼ cup of panko bread crumbs
- 1 teaspoon of salt-free Cajun seasoning
- 1 pound of catfish fillets

Directions:

1. Heat oven to 450° F
2. Use cooking spray to spray a non-stick baking sheet
3. Using a bowl, beat the egg white until very soft peaks are formed. Don't over-beat
4. Use a sheet of wax paper and place the flour over it
5. Using a different sheet of wax paper to combine and mix the cornmeal, panko and the Cajun seasoning

6. Cut the catfish fillet into four pieces, then dip the fish in the flour, shaking off the excess
7. Dip coated fish in the egg white, rolling into the cornmeal mixture
8. Place the fish on the baking pan. Repeat with the remaining fish fillets
9. Use cooking spray to spray over the fish fillets. Bake for about 10 to 12 minutes or until the sides of the fillets become browned and crisp

Nutrients Per Serving: Calories 250, Protein 22g, Carbohydrates 19g, Fat 10g, Cholesterol 53mg, Sodium 124mg, Potassium 401mg, Phosphorus 262mg, Fiber 1.2g

Tips:

- You can also use other recommended salt-free Cajun seasonings such as Andy Roo's The Stuff With No Salt, Mrs. Dash Extra Spicy seasoning or Benoit's spicy salt-free Cajun seasoning
- Panko can be found in most Asian markets and supermarkets, which is used for coating fried foods. In its absence, you can use unseasoned dry bread crumbs

Cilantro-Lime Cod

Suitable For: CKD non-dialysis, dialysis, and diabetes

Preparation Time: 10 minutes; **Cooking Time:** 35 minutes; **Servings:** 4; **Serving Size:** one 3-ounce fillet

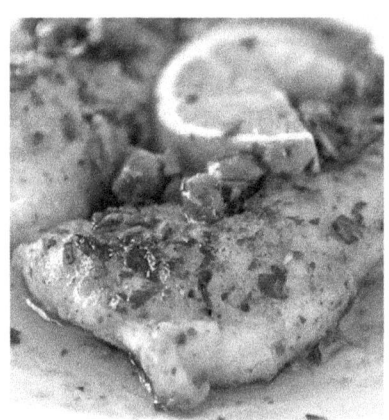

Ingredients:

- ½ cup of mayonnaise
- ½ cup of fresh chopped cilantro
- 2 tablespoon of lime juice
- 1 pound of cod fillets

Directions:

1. Combine and mix the mayonnaise, cilantro, and lime juice in a medium bowl, remove ¼ cup to another bowl and put aside. To be served as fish sauce

2. Spread the remaining mayonnaise mixture over the cod fillets
3. Use cooking spray to spray a large skillet, then heat over medium-high heat
4. Place in the cod fillets, and cook for about 8 minutes or until the fish becomes firm and moist, turning just once
5. Serve with the ¼ cilantro-lime sauce

Nutrients Per Serving: Calories 292, Protein 20g, Carbohydrates 1g, Fat 23g, Cholesterol 57mg, Sodium 228mg, Potassium 237mg, Phosphorus 128mg, Calcium 14mg

Tips:

- The cilantro can be substituted for ¼-cup of chopped fresh dill weed

Shrimp Quesadilla

Suitable For: CKD non-dialysis, dialysis, and diabetes

Preparation Time: 15 minutes; **Cooking Time:** 10 minutes; **Servings:** 2; **Serving Size:** 4 pieces

Ingredients:

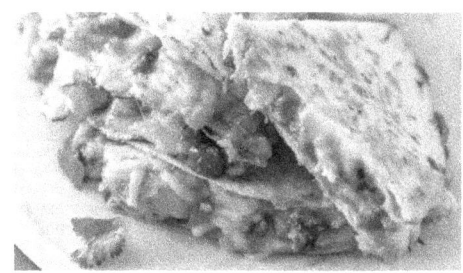

- 5 ounces of raw shrimp

- 2 tablespoons of cilantro
- 1 tablespoon of lemon juice
- ¼ teaspoon of ground cumin
- ⅛ teaspoon of cayenne pepper
- 2 flour burrito-sized tortillas
- 2 tablespoons of sour cream
- 4 teaspoons of salsa
- 2 tablespoons of shredded jalapeno cheddar cheese

Directions:

1. Peel the shrimp, rinse, and then cut into pieces of bite-size. Dice the cilantro
2. Use a zip-lock bag to combine and mix the cilantro, lemon juice, cumin, and cayenne pepper to make the marinade. Add the pieces of shrimp and put aside to marinate for about 5 minutes
3. Heat a skillet over medium heat and add the shrimp with the marinade. Stir-fry for about 1 to 2 minutes or until the shrimp is orange in color. Remove the skillet from heat and spoon out the shrimp, leaving marinade
4. Add the sour cream to the skillet with the leftover marinade. Stir to mix
5. Use a large skillet or microwave to heat the tortillas, then spread two teaspoons of salsa over each tortilla. Top with ½ of the shrimp mixture, sprinkling with one tablespoon of cheddar cheese

6. Spoon out one tablespoon of the sour cream mixture from step 4 on top of the shrimp, fold the tortilla into half, turning over in skillet to heat, then remove from the pan. Repeat the same process with the second tortilla and with the remaining shrimp, cheese and marinade
7. Cut each of the tortillas into four pieces, and serve

Nutrients Per Serving: Calories 318, Protein 20g, Carbohydrates 26g, Fat 15g, Cholesterol 118mg, Sodium 398mg, Potassium 276mg, Phosphorus 243mg, Fiber 1.2g

Chapter 8

Salad

Beet and Cucumber Salad

Suitable For: CKD non-dialysis, dialysis, and diabetes

Preparation Time: 10 minutes; **Cooking Time:** 10 minutes; **Servings:** 6; **Serving Size:** ¾ cup

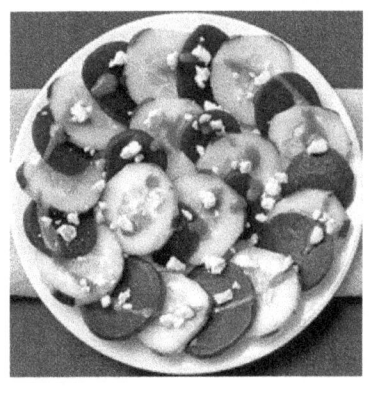

Ingredients:

- 1 cucumber
- 15 ounces of canned low-sodium sliced beets
- 4 teaspoons of balsamic vinegar
- 2 teaspoons of canola oil
- 2 tablespoons of Gorgonzola cheese

Directions:

1. Thinly slice the cucumber
2. Place the slices of beet on a serving plate
3. Layer the slices of cucumber over the beet slices
4. Drizzle layered beet slices with vinegar and oil
5. Sprinkle drizzled beet slices with Gorgonzola cheese

Nutrients Per Serving: Calories 74, Protein 1g, Carbohydrates 13g, Fat 2g, Cholesterol 2mg, Sodium 93mg, Potassium 207mg, Phosphorus 37mg, Fiber 1.7g

Tips:

- Gorgonzola cheese is a blue cheese Italian made, and high in sodium hence, a little amount is used for this recipe
- The beets should be chilled before the recipe is prepared

Chicken Apple Crunch Salad

Suitable For: CKD non-dialysis, dialysis, and diabetes

Preparation Time: 30 minutes; **Cooking Time:** 0 minutes; **Servings:** 4; **Serving Size:** ¾ cup

Ingredients:

- 2 cups of cooked chicken
- 1 cup of Gala apple
- ½ cup of celery

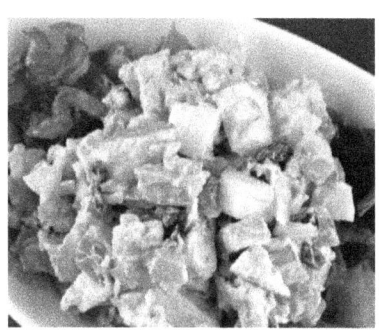

- 2 tablespoons of scallions
- ¼ cup of dark raisins
- ⅓ cup of low-fat mayonnaise
- 1 tablespoon of low-fat sour cream

- 1 teaspoon of lemon juice
- ¼ teaspoon of cinnamon
- ¼ teaspoon of black pepper

Directions:

1. Cube the cooked chicken, dice the apple and celery, and chop the scallions
2. Use a large salad bowl to combine and mix the chicken, apple, celery, scallions, and raisins
3. Whisk together the mayonnaise, lemon juice, sour cream, cinnamon, and black pepper. Pour on top of the chicken apple mixture and toss
4. Store in the refrigerator to chill before serving

Nutrients Per Serving: Calories 244, Protein 21g, Carbohydrates 13g, Fat 12g, Cholesterol 64mg, Sodium 221mg, Potassium 350mg, Phosphorus 158mg, Fiber 1.5g

Tips:

- The raisins can be excluded to reduce the potassium level to 270 mg per serving

Homestyle Macaroni Salad

Suitable For: CKD non-dialysis, dialysis, and diabetes

Preparation Time: 1 hr; **Cooking Time:** 15 minutes; **Servings:** 14; **Serving Size:** ½ cup

Ingredients:

- 8 ounces of uncooked macaroni
- ½ cup of celery
- ¼ cup of red onion
- ¼ cup of red bell pepper
- ½ tablespoon of jalapeno pepper
- ¾ cup of mayonnaise
- 1 tablespoon of cider vinegar
- 2 tablespoons of fresh chives
- ½ teaspoon of salt (or exclude to reduce sodium)
- ¼ teaspoon of black pepper

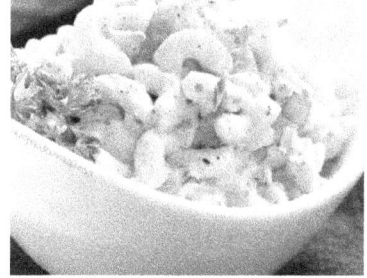

Directions:

1. Cook the pasta based on the package directions, move to a colander, and rinse with cold water. Drain and put aside
2. Finely chop the celery, red onion, bell pepper, and the jalapeno pepper

3. Combine and mix the remaining ingredients in a large bowl until it blends properly. Add the pasta, then toss to coat
4. Store in the refrigerator to chill for about 1 hour before serving

Nutrients Per Serving: Calories 173, Protein 3g, Carbohydrates 15g, Fat 11g, Cholesterol 5mg, Sodium 182mg, Potassium 63mg, Phosphorus 36mg, Fiber 0.6g

Gelatin Salad with Cottage Cheese and Pineapple

Suitable For: CKD non-dialysis, dialysis, and diabetes

Preparation Time: 1hr 30 minutes; **Cooking Time:** 15 minutes; **Servings:** 10; **Serving Size:** ½ cup

Ingredients:

- ½ cup of celery
- 20 ounces of canned and crushed pineapple, packed in juice
- 1 packet Knox of original unflavored gelatin
- ⅓ cup of lime juice
- ½ cup of low-fat milk
- 2 cups of cottage cheese

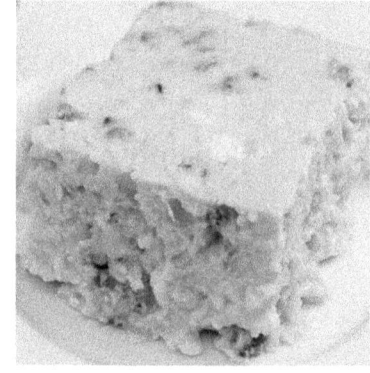

Directions:

1. Finely dice the celery
2. Drain the juice from the pineapple into a pan, then bring to a boil. Remove from heat
3. Pour the gelatin into the juice, stir until it is dissolved, and then stir into the lime juice
4. Stir mixture from step 3 into the pineapple, milk, cottage cheese, and celery.
5. Pour the mixture into a 9 x 13- inch dish and refrigerate, stirring every 15 minutes to mix and combine the ingredients evenly or until the gelatin starts to set
6. Chill for about 1 hour before serving

Nutrients Per Serving: Calories 81, Protein 6g, Carbohydrates 12g, Fat 1g, Cholesterol 6mg, Sodium 150mg, Potassium 167mg, Phosphorus 85mg, Fiber 0.6g

Fruited Curry Chicken Salad

Suitable For: CKD non-dialysis, dialysis, and diabetes

Preparation Time: 45 minutes; **Cooking Time:** 0 minutes; **Servings:** 8; **Serving Size:** 1 cup

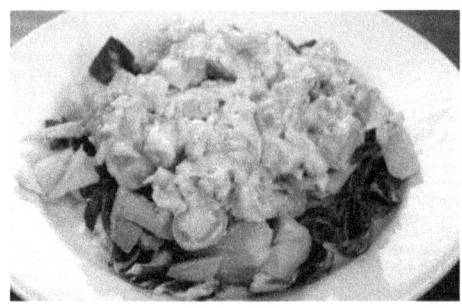

Ingredients:

- 4 cooked skinless and boneless chicken breasts
- 1 stalk of celery
- ½ cup of onion
- 1 medium-sized apple
- ¼ cup of seedless red grapes
- ¼ cup of seedless green grapes
- ½ cup of canned water chestnuts
- ⅛ teaspoon of black pepper
- ½ teaspoon of curry powder
- ¾ cup of mayonnaise

Directions:

1. Dice the chicken and chop the celery, onion, and apple. Also, drain and chop the water chestnuts
2. Combine and mix in a large bowl, the chicken, celery, apple, grapes, onion, water chestnuts, pepper, curry powder, and mayonnaise. Toss all ingredients together, then serve or chill for later

Nutrients Per Serving: Calories 238, Protein 14g, Carbohydrates 6g, Fat 18g, Cholesterol 44mg, Sodium 162mg, Potassium 200mg. Phosphorus 115mg, Fiber 1.1g

Ambrosia Salad with Marshmallow

Suitable For: CKD non-dialysis, dialysis, and diabetes

Preparation Time: 1hr 10 minutes; **Cooking Time:** 0 minutes; **Servings:** 4; **Serving Size:** ⅔ cup

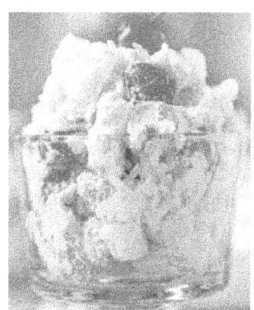

Ingredients:

- 8 ounces of canned crushed pineapple in juice
- 11 ounces of canned mandarin oranges
- ½ cup of mini marshmallows
- ¼ cup of sour cream
- 2 tablespoons of flaked coconut
- 8 maraschino cherries

Directions:

1. Properly drain pineapple and oranges
2. Use a bowl to combine and mix the remaining ingredients
3. Serve immediately or refrigerate for 1 hour to chill before serving

Nutrients Per Serving: Calories 127, Protein 1g, Carbohydrates 24g, Fat 3g, Cholesterol 6mg, Sodium 31mg, Potassium 127mg, Phosphorus 26mg, Fiber 1g

Rotini Pasta Salad

Suitable For: CKD non-dialysis, and diabetes

Preparation Time: 20 minutes; **Cooking Time:** 10 minutes; **Servings:** 8; **Serving Size:** ½ cup

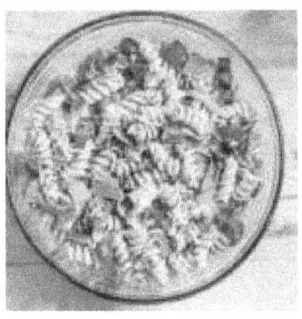

Ingredients:

- 4 ounces of uncooked rotini pasta, uncooked
- 1-¼ of cups onion

- 4 large eggs
- 1 medium-sized cucumber
- ½ cup of mayonnaise
- ½ teaspoon of black pepper
- 1 tablespoon of dry mustard
- ⅓ teaspoon of salt (or exclude to reduce sodium)
- 1 teaspoon of prepared mustard
- ½ cup of sugar
- ⅓ cup of vinegar

Directions:

1. Cook the rotini based on the instruction directions on the package, omit salt, drain and rinse
2. Hard boil the eggs, allow to cool, then peel
3. Chop the onion, eggs, and dice the cucumber
4. Combine and mix the rotini, onion, eggs, pepper, and cucumber in a large bowl
5. Combine the remaining ingredients to prepare the dressing
6. Add the homemade dressing to the pasta. Mix properly
7. Store in the refrigerator to chill before serving

Nutrients Per Serving: Calories 260, Protein 6g, Carbohydrates 28g, Fat 14g, Cholesterol 111mg, Sodium 193mg, Potassium 172mg, Phosphorus 87mg, Fiber 1.5g

Spinach-Mandarin Salad

Suitable For: CKD non-dialysis, dialysis, and diabetes

Preparation Time: 20 minutes; **Cooking Time:** 0 minutes; **Servings:** 8; **Serving Size:** 1 cup

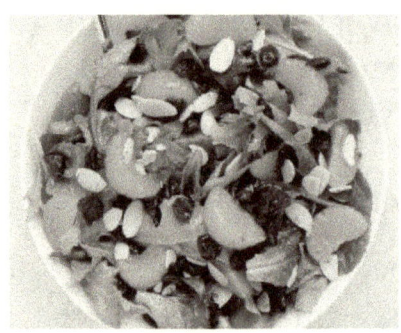

Ingredients:

- 2 cups of fresh spinach
- ½ cup of dried sweetened cranberries
- 5-ounce can of drained water chestnuts
- 1 cup of mandarin oranges
- 1 medium-sized apple
- ¼ cup of crunchy chow mein noodles
- 1 teaspoon of black pepper
- ¼ cup of vinaigrette salad dressing

Directions:

1. Drain the water chestnuts and oranges. Cut the apple into wedges

2. Using a 1-quart serving bowl, place in the washed and drained spinach, then spread on top, the dried cranberries
3. Add the water chestnuts, apple wedges, chow mein noodles, and the mandarin oranges
4. Sprinkle pepper over the top, then cover and store in the refrigerator to chill
5. Use ¼-cup of vinaigrette salad dressing to slightly toss over the mixture from step 4, then serve.

Nutrients Per Serving: Calories 157, Protein 2g, Carbohydrates 31g, Fat 4g, Cholesterol 0mg, Sodium 145mg, Potassium 232mg, Phosphorus 32mg, Fiber 2.9g

Tip:

- Leaf lettuce can be used as a substitute for the spinach, or you can use both

Turkey Waldorf Salad

Suitable For: CKD non-dialysis, dialysis, and diabetes

Preparation Time: 20 minutes; **Cooking Time:** 0 minutes; **Servings:** 6; **Serving Size:** ½ cup

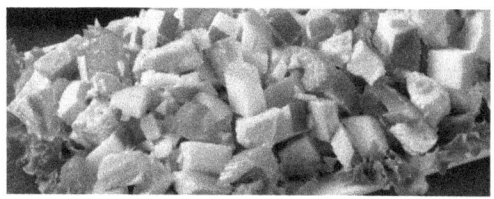

Ingredients:

- 12 ounces of unsalted and cooked turkey breast
- 3 medium-sized red apples
- 1 cup of celery
- ½ cup of onion
- ¼ cup of mayonnaise
- 2 tablespoons of apple juice

Directions:

1. Cut the turkey into cubes, dice the celery and apples and chop the onion
2. Combine and mix the turkey, apple, celery, and onion in a medium-sized bowl
3. Add the mayonnaise and apple juice, stirring properly until it is well mixed
4. Chill in the refrigerate until ready to serve

Nutrients Per Serving: Calories 200, Protein 17g, Carbohydrates 8g, Fat 11g, Cholesterol 60mg, Sodium 128mg, Potassium 296mg, Phosphorus 136mg, Fiber 1.9g

Tabbouleh Salad

Suitable For: CKD non-dialysis, dialysis, and diabetes

Preparation Time: 1hr 45 minutes; **Cooking Time:** 0 minutes; **Servings:** 8; **Serving Size:** ¾ cup

Ingredients:

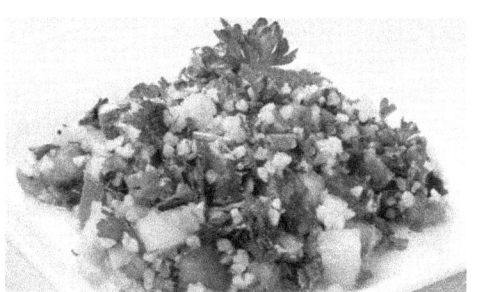

- ½ cup of dry bulgur
- 1 medium-sized tomato
- 1 medium-sized cucumber
- 1 bunch of green onions
- 2 bunches of parsley
- ½ bunch of mint
- ½ cup of olive oil
- 3 lemons
- ½ teaspoon of salt (or exclude to reduce sodium)
- ½ teaspoon of black pepper

Directions:

1. Wash and drain the bulgur, then place it in a large bowl. Pour ½ cup of boiling water on top of the bulgur, cover and set aside for 30 minutes
2. Dice the tomato, chop the peeled cucumber, parsley, green onions, and mint
3. Add the vegetables to the bulgur, stirring properly
4. Extract the lemon juice and add alongside the olive oil, salt, and pepper to the bulgur mixture
5. Before serving, set the salad at room temperature for 1 hour so that the lemon juice and olive oil is absorbed

Nutrients Per Serving: Calories 182, Protein 2g, Carbohydrates 12g, Fat 14g, Cholesterol 0mg, Sodium 160mg, Potassium 265mg, Phosphorus 53mg, Fiber 3.0g

Tips:

- Tabbouleh salad can be eaten with lettuce leaves or tender grape leaves

Chapter 9

Poultry and Meat Mains

Apple Spice Pork Chops

Suitable For: Dialysis and diabetes

Preparation Time: 10 minutes; **Cooking Time:** 35 minutes; **Servings:** 4; **Serving Size:** 1 pork chop, apples, and sauce

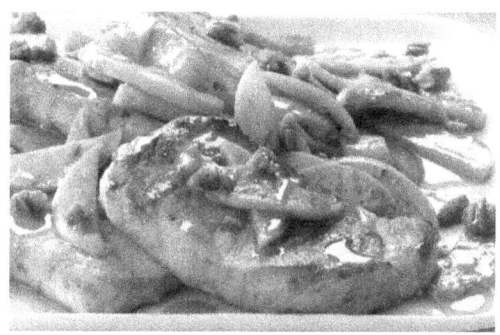

Ingredients:

- 1 pound of pork chops
- 2 tablespoons of unsalted butter
- ¼ cup of brown sugar
- ¼ teaspoon of salt (or exclude to reduce sodium)
- ¼ teaspoon of pepper
- ¼ teaspoon of nutmeg
- ¼ teaspoon of cinnamon
- 2 medium tart of apples

Directions:

1. Preheat oven to broil
2. Peel, and slice the apples
3. Broil the pork chops in the oven for about 4 to 5 minutes on both sides
4. Use a skillet to melt in the butter, stirring in the brown sugar, salt, nutmeg, cinnamon, pepper, and apples
5. Cover and cook until the apples become tender and the sauce starts to thicken
6. Spoon out the sauce over the cooked chops and serve

Nutrients Per Serving: Calories 306, Protein 22g, Carbohydrates 21g, Fat 16g, Cholesterol 88mg, Sodium 192mg, Potassium 473mg, Phosphorus 194mg, Fiber 1.2g

Tips:

- Marinate the pork chops in the apple juice, pepper, and chopped garlic for additional flavor
- Hot skillet can also be used to cook the pork chops instead of broiling. To do this, simply brush the chops with oil and cook for about 5 minutes on each side

Beef Burritos

Suitable For: CKD non-dialysis, dialysis, and diabetes

Preparation Time: 25 minutes; **Cooking Time:** 20 minutes; **Servings:** 6; **Serving Size:** 1 burrito

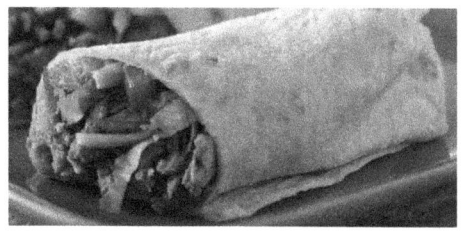

Ingredients:

- ¼ cup of onion
- ¼ cup of green pepper
- 1 pound of lean ground beef
- ¼ cup of low-sodium tomato puree
- ¼ teaspoon of black pepper
- ¼ teaspoon of ground cumin
- 6 burrito size flour tortillas

Directions:

1. Chop the onion and green pepper
2. Brown the ground beef in a medium skillet, and drain on paper towels
3. Spray the skillet with a non-stick cooking spray, then add the onion and green pepper. Cook for

about 3 to 5 minutes or until the vegetables become softened
4. Add the beef, tomato puree, cumin, and the black pepper to the onion and pepper mixture. Mix properly and cook over low heat for about 3 to 5 minutes
5. Divide beef mixture among the tortillas and rolling tortilla over burrito style. Make sure both ends are first folded so that the mixture doesn't fall off

Nutrients Per Serving: Calories 265, Protein 15g, Carbohydrates 31g, Fat 9g, Cholesterol 37mg, Sodium 341mg, Potassium 302mg, Phosphorus 171mg, Fiber 1.6g

Herb-Roasted Pork Tenderloin

Suitable For: CKD non-dialysis, dialysis, and diabetes

Preparation Time: 1hr 45 minutes; **Cooking Time:** 0 minutes; **Servings:** 7; **Serving Size:** 3 ounces

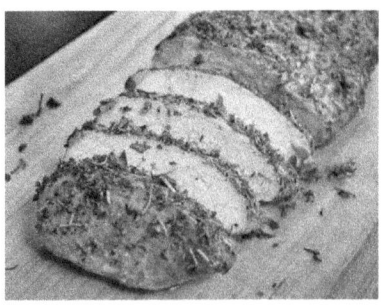

Ingredients:

- 2 garlic cloves
- 1 teaspoon of dried rosemary
- 1 teaspoon of dried thyme
- 1 teaspoon of dried basil
- 1 teaspoon of dried parsley
- 2 teaspoons of black pepper
- 2 tablespoons of Dijon mustard
- 2 (12-ounce) pork tenderloins
- 1½ tablespoons of vegetable oil

Directions:

1. Mince the garlic cloves, then add in a small bowl alongside the spices and mustard. Mix thoroughly
2. Rub the mixture of herb evenly over the pork tenderloins. Cover and refrigerate for about 2 hours
3. Preheat oven to 400° F
4. Use a large skillet to heat oil over medium-high heat. Place the tenderloins inside the heated oil and brown all the sides. Remove from skillet and place onto a baking dish without making contact with each other.
5. Bake tenderloins for about 20 minutes or until 160° F (medium) to 170° F (well done) is registered on the meat thermometer

6. Set the tenderloins aside to rest for about 10 to 15 minutes before carving. This will help distribute the juices throughout the meat

Nutrients Per Serving: Calories 178, Protein 24g, Carbohydrates 1g, Fat 8g, Cholesterol 67mg, Sodium 160mg, Potassium 401mg, Phosphorus 230mg, Fiber 0.4g

Tips:

- If you are on a low protein diet, reduce the serving size to match your meal plan

Asian Orange Chicken

Suitable For: CKD non-dialysis, dialysis, and diabetes

Preparation Time: 2hr 20 minutes; **Cooking Time:** 35 minutes; **Servings:** 4; **Serving Size:** ¼ of recipe

Ingredients:

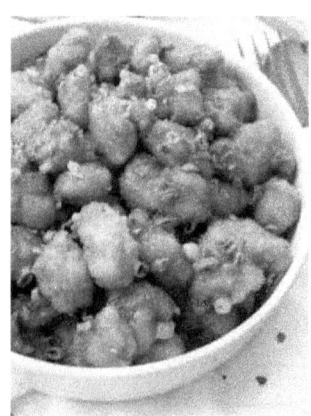

- 1¾ cups of water
- 2 tablespoons of orange juice
- ¼ cup of lemon juice
- ⅓ cup of unseasoned rice vinegar
- 2 tablespoons of reduced-sodium soy sauce

- 1 tablespoon of orange zest
- ⅓ cup packed of brown sugar
- ½ teaspoon of fresh ginger root
- 1 garlic clove
- 2 tablespoons of green onion
- ¼ teaspoon of red pepper flakes
- ½ pound of boneless, and skinless chicken breasts
- 2½ tablespoons of cornstarch
- 3 tablespoons of olive oil

Directions:

1. Mince the ginger root and garlic, and chop the green onion
2. Pour 1½ cups of water, lemon juice, orange juice, rice vinegar, and soy sauce into a saucepan and heat over medium-high heat. Stir in the orange zest, ginger, brown sugar, garlic, chopped onion, and the red pepper flakes, then bring to a boil. Remove from the heat, and allow to cool for about 10 to 15 minutes
3. Cut the chicken into ½ -inch pieces and place them into a sealable plastic bag. Pour 1 cup of the sauce from step 2 into the bag, reserve the rest of the sauce, seal the bag, and refrigerate for about 2 hours
4. Use a large skillet to heat olive oil over medium heat, then place the marinated chicken inside the skillet, browning each side. Drain over paper towels and set aside

5. Clean out the skillet, add in the remaining sauce from step 3, and bring to a boil over medium-high heat. Mix the cornstarch and the remaining cups of water, and stir into the sauce. Reduce the heat to medium-low, and add the pieces of chicken, then simmer for about 5 minutes. Stir occasionally
6. Cut into four portions and serve hot

Nutrients Per Serving: Calories 242, Protein 14g, Carbohydrates 19g, Fat 12g, Cholesterol 37mg, Sodium 340mg, Potassium 240mg, Phosphorus 118mg, Fiber 0.4g

Tips:

- To complete the meal, serve with steamed rice
- Chicken breast can be substituted for turkey cutlets, pork loin, or chicken thigh meat

Garlic Chicken with Balsamic Vinegar

Suitable For: Dialysis and diabetes

Preparation Time: 5 minutes; **Cooking Time:** 25 minutes; **Servings:** 4; **Serving Size:** 1 chicken breast

Ingredients:

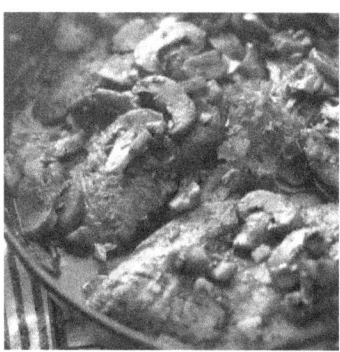

- 4 boneless, and skinless chicken breasts
- 1 teaspoon of fresh ground black pepper
- 1 tablespoon of olive oil
- 8 peeled garlic cloves
- ¾ cup of white button mushrooms, sliced
- ¼ cup of balsamic vinegar
- ¾ cup of low-sodium chicken broth
- 1 bay leaf
- ¼ teaspoon of thyme leaves
- 1 tablespoon of cornstarch

Directions:

1. Wash the chicken breasts, trim excess fat, and coat each side with pepper
2. Use a non-stick skillet and heat the olive oil medium-high heat. Cook for about 3 minutes or until it is browned
3. Add in the garlic, spread the mushrooms over, and turn the chicken around to prevent it from sticking to the mushroom. Cook for about 3 minutes
4. Mix the balsamic vinegar, low-sodium chicken broth, thyme leaves, cornstarch and the bay leaf in a small bowl

5. Add the mixture to the skillet with chicken, and stir until the sauce is thickened
6. Cover and cook for about 10 minutes over medium-low heat
7. Remove the bay leaf and garlic, and serve with rice or pasta

Nutrients Per Serving: Calories 211, Protein 30g, Carbohydrates 7g, Fat 7g, Cholesterol 73mg, Sodium 88mg, Potassium 337mg, Phosphorus 230mg, Fiber 0.5g

Turkey Breast with Cranberry Gravy

Suitable For: CKD non-dialysis, dialysis, and diabetes

Preparation Time: 10 minutes; **Cooking Time:** 4 hrs; **Servings:** 6; **Serving Size:** 2½ounces turkey, ⅓ cup vegetables, ¼ cup cranberry gravy

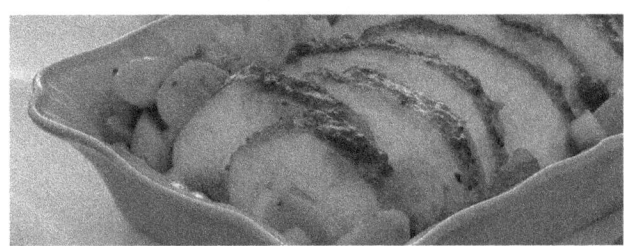

Ingredients:

- ¼ cup of onion
- ⅓ cup of celery
- 2 cups of carrots

- 18 ounces of boneless, skinless turkey breast
- 1 teaspoon of poultry seasoning
- ½ teaspoon of chicken bouillon granules
- 1 cup of cranberry sauce

Directions:

1. Dice the onion, and slice the celery and carrots
2. Spray a slow cooker with a non-stick cooking spray, place in the turkey breast, sprinkling with poultry seasoning and bouillon granules
3. Spoon out the cranberry sauce over the top, then add the vegetables from step 1
4. Cover the slow cooker, and cook for about 4 hours over high heat
5. Remove and slice the turkey breast, serving with the vegetables and cranberry gravy

Nutrients Per Serving: Calories 216, Protein 18g, Carbohydrates 25g, Fat 6g, Cholesterol 36mg, Sodium 183mg, Potassium 373mg, Phosphorus 187mg, Fiber 2.4g

Tips:

- You can substitute boneless turkey for a whole turkey breast
- A small portion of regular bouillon gives additional flavor. Controlling the portion helps

ensure the sodium content of a low-sodium diet is within the limits

Grilled Pineapple Chicken

Suitable For: Dialysis and diabetes

Preparation Time: 10 minutes; **Cooking Time:** 25 minutes; **Servings:** 4; **Serving Size:** 1 chicken breast

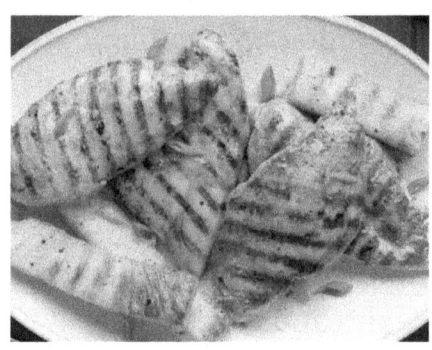

Ingredients:

- 1 cup of dry sherry
- 1 cup of pineapple juice
- 1 tablespoon of reduced-sodium soy sauce
- 1-¼ pound of skinless, bone-in chicken breast
- 4 pineapple rings

Directions:

1. Using a zip-lock bag, place in all the ingredients excluding the pineapple

2. Refrigerate and marinate overnight
3. Using an indoor or barbecue grill, place on top of the marinated chicken. Cook for about 15 to 20 minutes or until done, and discard the unused marinade
4. At the last few minutes of cooking, place the pineapple on top of the grill for about 2 minutes on both sides to heat
5. Serve each chicken breast, topped with the pineapple

Nutrients Per Serving: Calories 211, Protein 26g, Carbohydrates 20g, Fat 3g, Cholesterol 67mg, Sodium 215mg, Potassium 376mg, Phosphorus 198mg, Fiber 0.5g

Tips:

- Grilling is the recommended method of cooking and is tastier compared to when the chicken is oven-baked
- Cooking sherry and cooking wine both contain high sodium levels; hence, don't substitute the dry sherry in this recipe for either of the two

Chicken Enchiladas

Suitable For: CKD non-dialysis, dialysis, and diabetes

Preparation Time: 30 minutes; **Cooking Time:** 30 minutes; **Servings:** 6; **Serving Size:** 1 enchilada

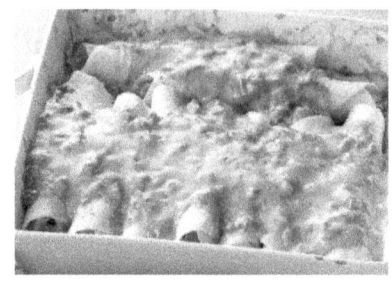

Ingredients:

- 10 ounces of boneless and skinless chicken breasts
- 1 packet of reduced-sodium taco sauce mix
- ⅔ cup of water
- 1 cup of diced red bell pepper
- 6 (6-inch) corn tortillas
- 6 tablespoons of sour cream

Directions:

1. Preheat oven to 350° F
2. Cut the chicken into strips and cook over medium-high heat with a skillet
3. Mix the taco sauce in a small bowl with ⅔ cup of water
4. Add in the red bell pepper alongside ⅓ cup of the taco sauce into the skillet. Cook until the chicken is ready
5. Using a baking dish, spray with a non-stick cooking spray
6. To prepare the enchiladas, spoon out the chicken and pepper mixture over the tortilla and roll up,

then place each of the enchiladas into the baking dish to hold the rolled shape. Pour the remainder of the taco sauce over the top
7. Bake the enchiladas for about 5 to 7 minutes or until the edges start to brown
8. Top each of the enchiladas with one tablespoon of sour cream, and serve

Nutrients Per Serving: Calories 169, Protein 14g, Carbohydrates 17g, Fat 5g, Cholesterol 37mg, Sodium 367mg, Potassium 215mg, Phosphorus 184mg, Fiber 1.8g

Tips:

- Packaged taco seasoning mix has a much lower potassium content than bottled or canned taco seasoning.
- Corn tortillas have a moderate phosphorus level. The phosphorous level of enchilada should be kept low by topping with sour cream instead of cheese

Roasted Leg of Lamb

Suitable For: CKD non-dialysis, dialysis, and diabetes

Preparation Time: 15 minutes; **Cooking Time:** 1hr 45 minutes; **Servings:** 10; **Serving Size:** 4 ounces

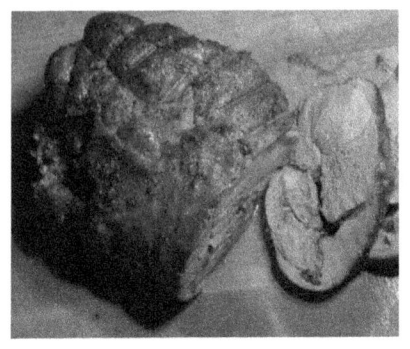

Ingredients:

- 4 tablespoons of unsalted butter
- 1 boneless leg of lamb (4½ pounds) rolled and tied
- ¼ cup of fresh rosemary leaves
- 2 garlic cloves
- 2 tablespoons of dried and crushed oregano leaves
- 1 teaspoon of salt (or exclude to reduce sodium)
- 1 teaspoon of black pepper
- ¼ cup of fresh lemon juice
- 1 cup of water

Directions:

1. Preheat oven to 325° F.
2. Set out the butter at room temperature
3. Wash and slightly trim fat from lamb. Put aside in a roasting pan
4. Chop the rosemary leaves and mince the garlic
5. Blend in a bowl the oregano, garlic, rosemary, salt, pepper and half of the soft butter
6. Cut the leg of lamb into slits, stuffing some of the herb and butter mixture inside the slits, and spreading the remaining herb and butter mixture over the lamb

7. Mix the lemon juice with the other half butter and pour over the lamb
8. Cover and bake for about 30 minutes for each pound
9. After 1 hour, add water to the drippings in the pan. Baste regularly until the meat is tender and browns properly.
10. For crisp skin, uncover the pan during the last half hour.

Nutrients Per Serving: Calories 318, Protein 30g, Carbohydrates 0g, Fat 22g, Cholesterol 118mg, Sodium 326mg or 114mg without salt, Potassium 394mg, Phosphorus 228mg, Fiber 0.5g

Tips:

- If you are on a low protein diet, reduce the serving size to match your meal plan or check with your dietitian

Cranberry Pork Chops

Suitable For: CKD non-dialysis, dialysis, and diabetes

Preparation Time: 20 minutes; **Cooking Time:** 45 minutes; **Servings:** 6; **Serving Size:** 1 pork chop and ½ cup rice

Ingredients:

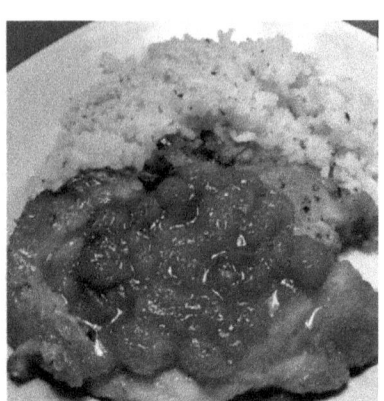

- 6 (4 ounces) boneless pork loin chops
- ¼ teaspoon of ground black pepper
- 2 teaspoons of cornstarch
- 1 cup of cranapple juice
- 2 teaspoons of honey
- ¾ cup of dried, sweetened cranberries
- 1 tablespoon of fresh minced tarragon
- 1 tablespoon of fresh minced parsley
- 3 cups of brown cooked rice

Directions:

1. Sprinkle pepper over the pork chops
2. Use a cooking spray to coat a large non-stick skillet, then cook the chops on each side for about 3 to 4 minutes over medium heat or until it is lightly browned
3. Remove the chops from the skillet and keep warm
4. Mix the cornstarch, juice, and honey in a small bowl until it becomes smooth, then add to the skillet. Stir to loosen browned bits

5. Add and stir in the cranberries, tarragon, and parsley, then bring to a boil. Cook for 2 minutes or until it is thickened and bubbly
6. Add the pork loins to the pan. Cover and reduce the heat, simmering for about 4 to 6 minutes or until the meat thermometer reads 160° F
9. Serve with hot brown rice

Nutrients Per Serving: Calories 397, Protein 25g, Carbohydrates 45g, Fat 13g, Cholesterol 64mg, Sodium 76mg, Potassium 410mg, Phosphorus 267mg, Fiber 2.7g

Tips:

- If you are on a low protein diet, reduce the serving size of the pork to match your meal plan

Chapter 10

Dessert

Apple Pie Bars

Suitable For: CKD non-dialysis, dialysis, and diabetes

Preparation Time: 25 minutes; **Cooking Time:** 40 minutes; **Servings:** 18; **Serving Size:** 1 bar, 3 x 3-inch

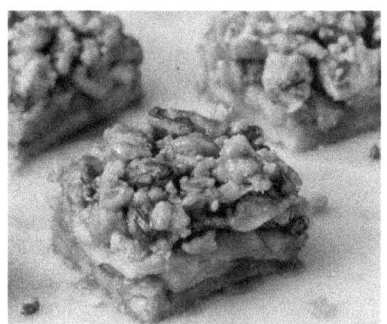

Ingredients:

- 2 medium-sized apples
- ¾ cup of unsalted melted butter
- 1 cup of granulated sugar
- 1 cup of sour cream
- 1 teaspoon of vanilla extract
- 1 teaspoon of baking soda
- ½ teaspoon of salt (or exclude to reduce sodium)
- 2 cups of all-purpose flour

- ½ cup of brown sugar
- 1 teaspoon of cinnamon
- 2 tablespoons of milk
- 1 cup of powdered sugar

Directions:

1. Preheat oven to 350° F
2. Peel and chop the apples
3. Together, cream ½ cup of butter and granulated sugar in a bowl
4. Stir in the sour cream, baking soda, vanilla, salt, flour, and the chopped apples
5. Transfer the batter onto a 9 x 13-inch greased baking pan
6. Combine and mix two tablespoons of butter, brown sugar and cinnamon in a small bowl, then sprinkle over the batter
7. Bake for about 35 to 40 minutes, then allow it cool completely
8. To make the icing, combine and mix two tablespoons of melted butter, powdered sugar, and milk, then drizzle over the top of the baked apple bar
9. Cut into 18 bars

Nutrients Per Serving: Calories 246, Protein 2g, Carbohydrates 35g, Fat 11g, Cholesterol 26mg, Sodium 140mg, Potassium 72mg, Phosphorus 27mg, Fiber 0.6g

Tips:

- If you have diabetes, you can substitute the granulated sugar for its alternative while also omitting the icing which will lower carbohydrate level to 19 grams per serving

Blueberry Peach Crisp

Suitable For: CKD non-dialysis, dialysis, and diabetes

Preparation Time: 10 minutes; **Cooking Time:** 45 minutes; **Servings:** 10; **Serving Size:** 1/10 of recipe

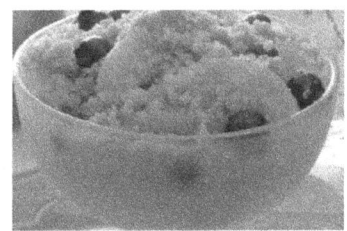

Ingredients:

- 7 medium-sized fresh peaches
- 1 cup of blueberries
- ¼ cup of granulated sugar
- 1 tablespoon of lemon juice
- ¾ cup of all-purpose flour
- ¾ cup of packed brown sugar
- ½ cup of butter

Directions:

1. Preheat oven to 375° F
2. Pit and slice the peaches into ¾- inch slices
3. Use a cooking spray to spray a 12 x 9-inch baking dish, then place the peach slices and blueberries on top of the dish
4. Sprinkle over the fruit, sugar and lemon juice
5. Use a small bowl to combine and mix the flour and brown sugar
6. Cut the butter into the flour mixture using two knives or pastry blender until it is crumbly. Sprinkle the crumbs on top of the fruit
7. Bake for about 45 minutes or until the fruit becomes soft and the crumbs are browned, then serve warm

Nutrients Per Serving: Calories 238, Protein 2g, Carbohydrates 35g, Fat 10g, Cholesterol 24mg, Sodium 76mg, Potassium 240mg, Phosphorus 36mg, Fiber 2.1g

Tips:

- If fresh peaches are unavailable, substitute with 4 cups of drained canned peach slices

Cherry Coffee Cake

Suitable For: CKD non-dialysis, dialysis, and diabetes

Preparation Time: 10 minutes; **Cooking Time:** 40 minutes; **Servings:** 24; **Serving Size:** 2 x 3-inch piece

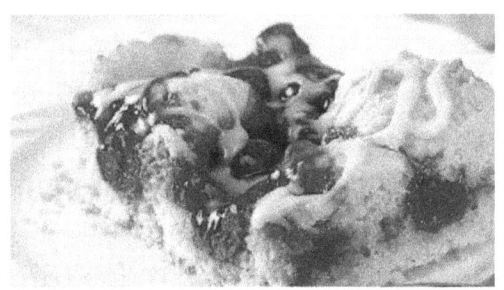

Ingredients:

- ½ cup of unsalted butter
- 2 eggs
- 1 cup of granulated sugar
- 1 cup of sour cream
- 1 teaspoon of vanilla
- 2 cups of all-purpose white flour
- 1 teaspoon of baking powder
- 1 teaspoon of baking soda
- 20 ounces of cherry pie filling

Directions:

1. Preheat the oven to 350° F
2. Set out the butter at room temperature to soften

3. Use a bowl to cream the butter, eggs, sour cream, sugar and vanilla
4. Combine and mix the flour, baking powder and baking soda in a separate bowl
5. Add the dry ingredients from step 4 to the creamed butter mixture. Mix properly, then pour the batter onto a greased 9 x 13-inch baking pan
6. Evenly spread the cherry pie filling over the batter
7. Bake for about 40 minutes or until it is golden brown

Nutrients Per Serving: Calories 204, Protein 3g, Carbohydrates 30g, Fat 8g, Cholesterol 43mg, Sodium 113mg, Potassium 72mg, Phosphorus 70mg, Fiber 0.5g

Tips:

- If you desire, replace the cherry filling with blueberry or raspberry pie filling
- If you have diabetes, substitute sugar for low sugar substitutes and use low-sugar cherry filling

Fruity Peach Crisp Dump

Suitable For: CKD non-dialysis, dialysis, and diabetes

Preparation Time: 10 minutes; **Cooking Time:** 30 minutes; **Servings:** 12; **Serving Size:** 1/12 of cake

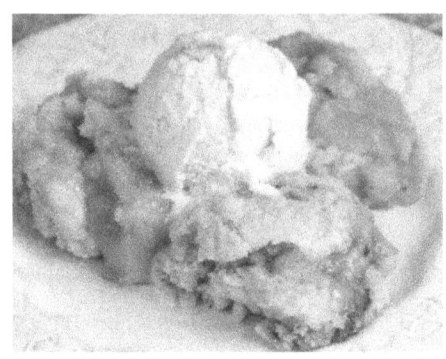

Ingredients:

- 40 ounces of sliced canned peaches
- Non-stick cooking spray
- 15.25 ounces of boxed yellow dry mix cake
- ½ cup of unsalted margarine

Directions:

1. Preheat oven to 350° F
2. Spray the cooking spray over a 9 x 13-inch cake pan
3. Dump two cans of undrained peaches onto the cake pan, spreading evenly
4. Evenly sprinkle the yellow cake mix on top of the fruit, and dot with margarine
5. Bake for about 30 minutes

Nutrients Per Serving: Calories 260, Protein 1g, Carbohydrates 44g, Fat 9g, Cholesterol 0mg, Sodium 292mg, Potassium 107mg, Phosphorus 140mg, Fiber 0.7g

Tips:

- Pineapple or any favorite canned fruit of yours can substitute the canned peaches
- If desired, you can serve with whipped topping
- If you have diabetes, reduce the serving size (if needed) to remain within your carbohydrate limit

Gingersnap Cookies

Suitable For: CKD non-dialysis, dialysis, and diabetes

Preparation Time: 10 minutes; **Cooking Time:** 1hr 10 minutes; **Servings:** 24; **Serving Size:** 2 cookies

Ingredients:

- 2 cups of all-purpose white flour
- 3 teaspoons of baking soda
- 1 teaspoon of ground cloves
- 1 teaspoon of ground ginger
- 1 teaspoon of ground cinnamon
- 1 stick of unsalted softened butter
- 1 cup of granulated sugar
- 1 egg
- 2 tablespoons of molasses

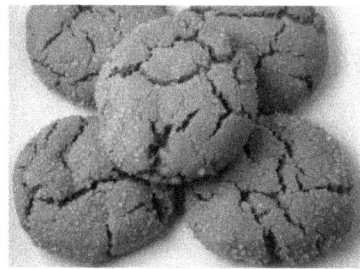

Directions:

1. Sift together, the flour, baking soda, ginger, cloves and cinnamon
2. Cream the butter using a mixer until it becomes light and fluffy, add sugar gradually, then blend in the egg and molasses
3. Pour in a little amount of the flour mixture at a time until a dough is formed
4. Cover and store in the refrigerator for 1 hour or overnight
5. Preheat oven to 350° F
6. Form the dough into a heaped teaspoon ball size, and place 2-inch apart on top a greased cookie sheet. Slightly flatten each ball
7. Bake for about 8 to 10 minutes, then cool on a wire rack
8. Make four dozen of cookies

Nutrients Per Serving: Calories 108, Protein 1g, Carbohydrates 17g, Fat 4g, Cholesterol 20mg, Sodium 162mg, Potassium 40mg, Phosphorus 14mg, Fiber 0.3g

Lemon Icebox Pie

Suitable For: CKD non-dialysis, dialysis, and diabetes

Preparation Time: 4hr 10 minutes; **Cooking Time:** 0 minutes; **Servings:** 8; **Serving Size:** ⅛ pie

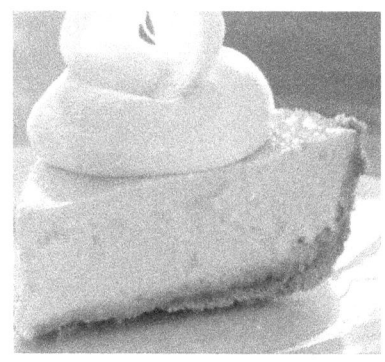

Ingredients:

- ½ cup of water
- 1 small packet of Knox unflavored gelatin
- 8 ounces of light sour cream
- 2½ cups of fat-free Reddi-Wip dairy whipped topping
- ¼ cup of lemon juice
- ⅓ cup of granulated sugar
- ¼ teaspoon of lemon extract
- 6 drops of yellow food coloring
- 1 graham (9-inch) cracker pie crust

Directions:

1. Dissolve the gelatin into ½ cup of boiling water, and allow it to stand for about five minutes
2. Combine and mix the sour cream, 2 cups of whipped topping, lemon juice, sugar, lemon extract, and food coloring. Stir in the dissolved gelatin
3. Pour the mixture into a pie shell, and store in the refrigerator for about 4 hours or until it is set
4. Cut into slices, topping each with one tablespoon of the remaining whipped topping

Nutrients Per Serving: Calories 253, Protein 4g, Carbohydrates 35g, Fat 11g, Cholesterol 13mg, Sodium 210mg, Potassium 116mg, Phosphorus 54mg, Fiber 0.5g

Strawberry Pavlova

Suitable For: CKD non-dialysis and dialysis

Preparation Time: 30 minutes; **Cooking Time:** 1hr 15 minutes; **Servings:** 8; **Serving Size:** ⅛ slice

Ingredients:

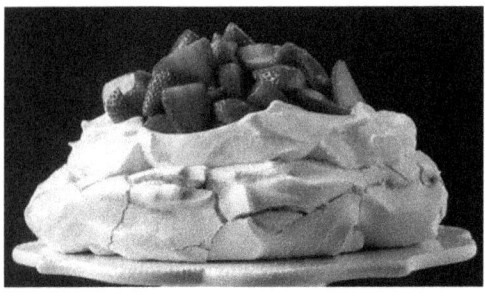

- 6 large egg white
- ⅛ teaspoon of salt (or exclude to reduce sodium)
- 2 cups and two tablespoons of granulated sugar
- 1½ teaspoons of vinegar
- 2½ teaspoons of vanilla extract
- 8 ounces of heavy whipping cream
- 4 cups of fresh sliced strawberries

Directions:

1. Preheat oven to 300º F.
2. Set out the egg white at room temperature; slice the strawberries and keep aside

3. Beat the egg white with salt until soft peaks are formed. Add 2 cups of sugar, one tablespoon at a time, and beat properly after each addition. Fold in the vinegar gently, adding 1½ teaspoons of vanilla
4. Use an 8-inch round, and ungreased cookie sheet to smooth in the mixture
5. Bake for about 45 minutes, then allow the shell to set for about 1 hour with the oven door closed. Remove from the oven, allowing it to cool completely
6. Add sugar, whipping cream, and the remaining 1 teaspoon of vanilla into a bowl, whipping with a mixer until it becomes stiff. Place the whipped cream in the freezer for about 10-15 minutes
7. Fill the top of the Pavlova shell from step 5 with the whipped topping and sliced berries

Nutrients Per Serving: Calories 355, Protein 4g, Carbohydrates 60g, Fat 11g, Cholesterol 39mg, Sodium 90mg, Potassium 175mg, Phosphorus 39mg, Fiber 1.0g

Tips:

- Due to high content in carbohydrate, this recipe is not recommended for people with diabetes

Snickerdoodles

Suitable For: CKD non-dialysis, dialysis, and diabetes

Preparation Time: 15 minutes; **Cooking Time:** 10 minutes; **Servings:** 24; **Serving Size:** 2 cookies

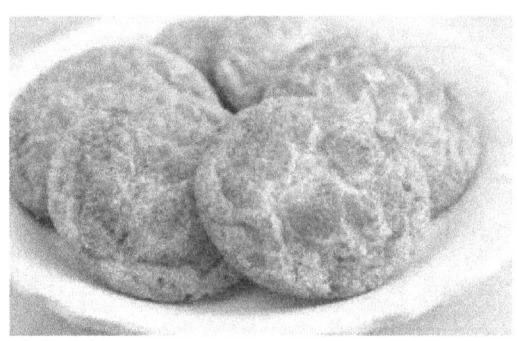

Ingredients:

- 2¾ cups of all-purpose white flour
- 1¾ cups of sugar (divided use)
- 1 cup of softened butter
- 2 eggs
- 2 teaspoons cream of tartar
- 1 teaspoon of baking soda
- 1 teaspoon of vanilla
- 1½ teaspoon of ground cinnamon

Directions:

1. Preheat oven to 400° F

2. Use a large bowl to combine and mix all the cookie ingredients, excluding the cinnamon and leaving out ¼ of the sugar
3. Using a small bowl, stir in the remaining sugar and the cinnamon
4. Form 1-inch of balls and roll into the sugar mixture
5. Use an ungreased cookie sheet to place in the dough balls, 2-inch apart
6. Bake for about 8 to 10 minutes or until it is browned

Nutrients Per Serving: Calories 185, Protein 2g, Carbohydrates 24g, Fat 9g, Cholesterol 39mg, Sodium 60mg, Potassium 66mg, Phosphorus 26mg, Fiber 0.5g

Bread Pudding

Suitable For: CKD non-dialysis, dialysis, and diabetes

Preparation Time: 15 minutes; **Cooking Time:** 40 minutes; **Servings:** 6; **Serving Size:** ½ cup

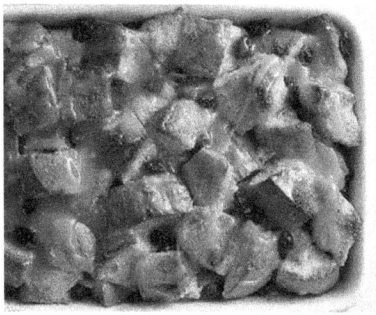

Ingredients:

- 2 large eggs
- 2 egg white
- 1½ cups of almond milk
- 2 tablespoons of honey
- 1 teaspoon of vanilla
- 2 tablespoons rum or 1 teaspoon rum extract
- 4 slices of raisin bread

Directions:

1. Preheat oven to 325º F
2. Use a non-stick cooking spray to spray an 8-inch round baking dish
3. Beat the eggs and egg white in a large mixing bowl until it is foamy. Beat in the almond milk, vanilla, honey, and the rum or rum extract
4. Cut the bread into cubes, stir into the egg mixture then spread over the baking dish
5. Bake for about 35 to 40 minutes or until it comes out clean when a knife is inserted at the center
6. Spoon out warm pudding into dishes to serve

Nutrients Per Serving: Calories 124, Protein 5g, Carbohydrates 19g, Fat 3g, Cholesterol 62mg, Sodium 148mg, Potassium 115mg, Phosphorus 59mg, Fiber 1.0g

Tips:

- You can substitute almond milk for unenriched rice milk. Always ensure you check the ingredient label for any milk or its substitute products, avoiding any with phosphate additives.

Frozen Fruit Delight

Suitable For: CKD non-dialysis, dialysis, and diabetes

Preparation Time: 3hr; **Cooking Time:** 0 minutes; **Servings:** 10; **Serving Size:** ½ cup

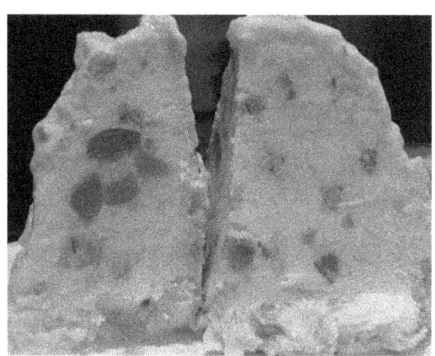

Ingredients:

- ⅓ cup of maraschino cherries
- 8 ounces of canned crushed pineapple
- 8 ounces of reduced-fat sour cream
- 1 tablespoon of lemon juice
- 1 cup of sliced strawberries
- ½ cup of sugar

- ⅛ teaspoon of salt
- 3 cups of Reddi-Wip dairy whipped topping

Directions:

1. Chop the cherries and drain the pineapple
2. Place all the ingredients into a medium-sized bowl except the whipped topping. Mix until well blended, then fold in the whipped topping.
3. Place the mixture into a freezable plastic container. Freeze for about 2 to 3 hours or until it is hardened

Nutrients Per Serving: Calories 133, Protein 1g, Carbohydrates 21g, Fat 5g, Cholesterol 21mg, Sodium 59mg, Potassium 99mg, Phosphorus 36mg, Calcium 47mg, Fiber 0.8g

Tips:

- Use ½ cup of Splenda granular sweetener to substitute the sugar if you have diabetes. This will reduce the carbohydrate content to 13g
- Fresh or frozen strawberries can be used for this recipe

Italian Tiramisu Cheesecake

Suitable For: CKD non-dialysis, dialysis, and diabetes

Preparation Time: 45 minutes; **Cooking Time:** 0 minutes; **Servings:** 10; **Serving Size:** 1/10 of recipe

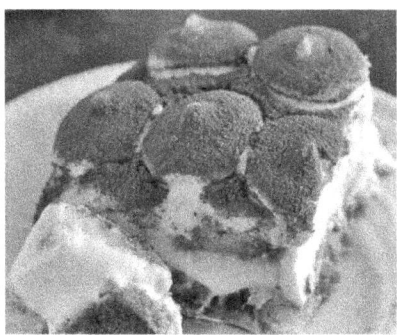

Ingredients:

- 10 ounces of prepared pound cake
- 12 ounces of regular cream cheese
- ½ cup of sugar
- 1 teaspoon of vanilla extract
- 2 tablespoons of unsweetened cocoa
- 1 ounce of semisweet finely grated chocolate
- 4 ounces of brewed espresso

Directions:

1. Cut the pound cake into ten even slices, and set aside
2. Mix the cream cheese, vanilla, and sugar in a bowl until it is smooth

3. Use a separate bowl to combine and mix the cocoa and grated chocolate, then set aside
4. Pour the espresso into a shallow dish
4. Dip the sides of 4 pieces of pound cake into the espresso, placing them in an 8 –inch loaf pan. Break the pieces up, if required to coat the bottom of the pan
5. Gently spread ⅓ of the cream cheese mixture over the cake layer in step 4, sprinkling with ⅓ of the cocoa mixture. Repeat procedure with the remaining slices of pound cake, and the cream cheese and cocoa mixture to make three layers
6. Refrigerate for about 2 hours, then cut into pieces of 10 and serve

Nutrients Per Serving: Calories 304, Protein 4g, Carbohydrates 27g, Fat 20g, Cholesterol 72mg, Sodium 196mg, Potassium 118mg, Phosphorus 85mg, Fiber 0.7g

Tips:

- To reduce carbohydrates and fat, rather than use sugar, use its substitute, and swap regular cream cheese with low-fat cream cheese. Serving size can also be adjusted to be smaller

Vanilla Lasagna

Suitable For: CKD non-dialysis, dialysis, and diabetes

Preparation Time: 12 hours; **Cooking Time:** 0 minutes; **Servings:** 15; **Serving Size:** One 3 x 2½ -inch piece

Ingredients:

- 4 containers of Snack Pack vanilla pudding
- 1 box honey graham crackers
- 13 ounces of fat-free Reddi Wip dairy dessert topping
- 1 cup of mini chocolate chip morsels

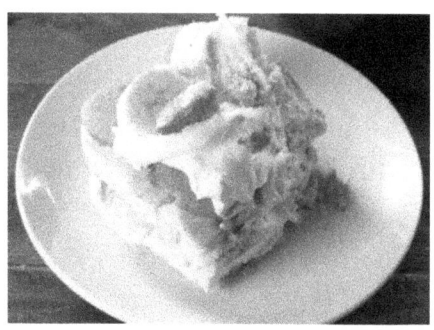

Directions:

1. Use a bowl to empty the vanilla pudding, then cut 3 cups of Reddi Wip into the bowl
2. Using a 9 x 13-inch pan, layer its bottom with graham crackers, and spread half of the pudding mixture over the crackers
3. Add another layer of the graham crackers over the pudding mixture, then spread the remaining pudding mixture over the crackers

4. Put the final layer of the graham crackers over the pudding mixture, and refrigerate overnight
5. Before serving, spray the top of the graham pudding mixture with the remaining Reddi Wip topping, then sprinkle the 1 cup of chocolate chip morsels over the top

Nutrients Per Serving: Calories 257, Protein 4g, Carbohydrates 40g, Fat 9g, Cholesterol 4mg, Sodium 188mg, Potassium 138mg, Phosphorus 91mg, Fiber 1.7g

Tips:

- It is best to prepare this recipe the night before when you want to serve it (about 12 hours)
- If you have diabetes, reduce the serving size to ½ the size recommended

Lemon Yogurt Parfait

Suitable For: CKD non-dialysis, dialysis, and diabetes

Preparation Time: 15 minutes; **Cooking Time:** 0 minutes; **Servings:** 4; **Serving Size:** 1 cup

Ingredients:

- 16 ounces of vanilla Greek yogurt
- 1 teaspoon of vanilla extract

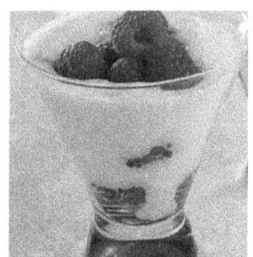

- 4 teaspoons of lemon juice
- ½ teaspoon of lemon zest
- ¾ cup of fat-free dairy whipped topping
- 1 cup of fresh raspberries

Directions:

1. Using a bowl, combine and mix the Greek yogurt, vanilla extract, lemon zest, and lemon juice until it becomes smooth, then fold in ½ cup of the dairy whipped topping
2. Divide the mixture into half, then further divide into four servings in parfait glasses. Top each serving with ¼ cup and two tablespoons of raspberries, and also topping each serving with the remaining yogurt mixture. Store in the refrigerator to chill
3. Before serving, top each parfait with one tablespoon of the remaining whipped topping and the remaining raspberries

Nutrients Per Serving: Calories 137, Protein 10g, Carbohydrates 22g, Fat 2g, Cholesterol 2mg, Sodium 45mg, Potassium 197mg, Phosphorus 145mg, Fiber 3g

Tips:

- You can substitute raspberries for strawberries or blueberries

Arroz Con Leche (Rice with Milk)

Suitable For: CKD non-dialysis, dialysis, and diabetes

Preparation Time: 10 minutes; **Cooking Time:** 20 minutes; **Servings:** 6; **Serving Size:** ½ cup

Ingredients:

- 1 cup of uncooked brown rice
- 2 cups of unsweetened almond milk
- 2 tablespoons of raisins

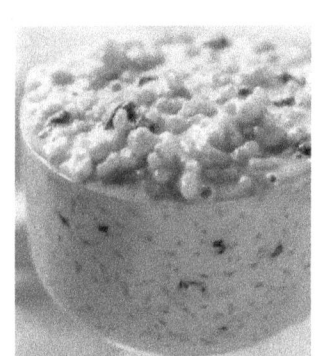

- ¼ cup of granulated sugar
- ¼ teaspoon of cinnamon
- 1 teaspoon of vanilla extract

Directions:

1. Rinse the rice then drain
2. Using a medium-sized saucepan, pour in the rice and add 1 cup water, then bring to a boil, cooking for about 10 minutes
3. Stir in the almond milk and raisins, and boil for an additional 10 minutes or until the rice is properly cooked
4. Remove from heat, stirring in the sugar, cinnamon, and vanilla. Mix properly and serve warm

Nutrients Per Serving: Calories 249, Protein 3g, Carbohydrates 37g, Fat 1g, Cholesterol 0mg, Sodium 60mg, Potassium 115mg, Phosphorus 52mg, Fiber 0.8g

Tips:

- Select a brand of unrefrigerated almond milk that has no phosphate additives
- Raisins are optional. However, when used, it should be limited as a result of the added potassium content

Bavarian Apple Torte

Suitable For: CKD non-dialysis, dialysis, and diabetes

Preparation Time: 30 minutes; **Cooking Time:** 35 minutes; **Servings:** 10; **Serving Size:** 1 slice

Ingredients:

- ½ cup of unsalted butter
- 1 cup of granulated sugar
- ¾ teaspoon of vanilla extract
- 1 cup of all-purpose white flour

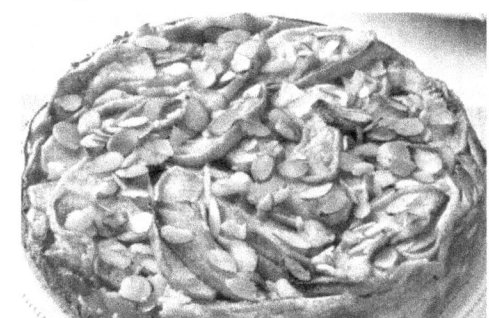

- 8 ounces of cream cheese
- 1 large egg
- ½ teaspoon of cinnamon
- 4 medium-sized apples
- ¼ cup of slivered almonds

Directions:

1. Preheat oven to 450° F
2. Set out the cream cheese to soften, then peel, and slice the apples
3. Altogether, cream the butter, ⅓ cup of sugar and ¼ teaspoon of vanilla extract, then fold in the flour to make the dough
5. Using a 9-inch springform pan, spread the dough on its bottom and sides
6. Using a medium-sized bowl, combine and mix the cream cheese with a ⅓ cup of sugar, then add the egg and a ½ teaspoon of vanilla. Mix properly until it is well blended. Pour the mixture over the crust from step 5
7. Combine and mix the last ⅓ cup of sugar and ½ teaspoon of cinnamon in another bowl, add the apples and toss until all are well coated
8. Spoon out the apple mixture over the cream cheese layer from step 6, and sprinkle with almonds
9. Bake at 450° F for about 10 minutes, then reduce the heat to 400° F and bake for an extra 25 minutes or until the center is set

10. Cool on a wire rack, and loosen torte from the rim of pan.
11. Before serving, cover and refrigerate for about 3 hours, storing any leftovers in the refrigerator

Nutrients Per Serving: Calories 340, Protein 4g, Carbohydrates 36g, Fat 20g, Cholesterol 72mg, Sodium 150mg, Potassium 130mg, Phosphorus 71mg, Fiber 1.6g

Tip:

- Fresh cranberries can be substituted for slivered almonds to reduce the phosphorus content to 53 mg per serving

Conclusion

Congratulations on having to transit the lines of this book from start to finish.

In this book, I have provided better insights into how the kidneys work, what could affect the functioning of the kidneys, the typical signs, and symptoms associated with kidney malfunctioning, the stages of kidney disease, and likewise, the changes that must be adhered to prevent further damage and eventual kidney failure— most of which centered around dietary choices. Because we are accustomed to everyday eating, it has become increasingly important to not only watch what we eat but also how we eat most especially, if you have CKD. Being able to manage your CKD is very vital to the long term sustainability and functionality of your kidneys. A renal diet, as explained in this book, is so significant that it provides you with better oversight of what to eat, what not to eat and also, how you eat – all of which is geared toward managing your CKD and delaying the progression of the disease. This book has provided you with most of the tools needed to get you started toward a prolonged kidney function by elaborating on a variety of handpicked low sodium, potassium, and phosphorus recipes that you can have for breakfast, as snacks and appetizers, soups and stews, vegetables, salads, meats, and desserts, coupled with the necessary nutritional information to guide your choices – which you can also use in adapting to your daily meal plans. Hence, it is my sincere desire that you found great value from this book.

Finally, I want you to take full responsibility for the health of your kidneys and overall wellbeing by incorporating what I have shared in this book into your daily dietary choices. I believe doing so would prevent further damage to your kidneys while also prolonging its ability to function healthily without the need for dialysis or transplant as it did for my patients.

On a lighter note, if you have found any benefit reading this book, I'd appreciate it if you could take some time to leave an honest review on the product page of this book. Reviews encourage other readers to give independent authors like myself a chance. They help more than I can describe. And trust me, I could use all the help you provide; thanks.

I wish you all the best on your journey toward health and wellness!

www.ingramcontent.com/pod-product-compliance
Lightning Source LLC
Chambersburg PA
CBHW031148020426
42333CB00013B/568